NOISE CONTROL

A Primer

A Singular Audiology Text
Jeffrey L. Danhauer, Ph.D.
Audiology Editor

NOISE CONTROL

A Primer

ALBERTO BEHAR, B.A.Sc., P.Eng.
Institute of Bioengineering
University of Toronto

MARSHALL CHASIN, M.Sc., Reg.CALPSO, Aud(C)
Department of Linguistics
University of Western Ontario

MARGARET CHEESMAN, Ph.D.
National Centre for Audiology
School of Communication Sciences and Disorders
University of Western Ontario

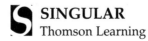

SINGULAR
Thomson Learning

Africa • Australia • Canada • Denmark • Japan • Mexico • New Zealand • Philippines
Puerto Rico • Singapore • Spain • United Kingdom • United States

NOTICE TO THE READER

Publisher does not warrant or guarantee any of the products described herein or perform any independent analysis in connection with any of the product information contained herein. Publisher does not assume, and expressly disclaims, any obligation to obtain and include information other than that provided to it by the manufacturer.

The reader is expressly warned to consider and adopt all safety precautions that might be indicated by the activities herein and to avoid all potential hazards. By following the instructions contained herein, the reader willingly assumes all risks in connection with such instructions.

The Publisher makes no representation or warranties of any kind, including but not limited to, the warranties of fitness for particular purpose or merchantability, nor are any such representations implied with respect to the material set forth herein, and the publisher takes no responsibility with respect to such material. The publisher shall not be liable for any special, consequential, or exemplary damages resulting, in whole or part, from the readers' use of, or reliance upon, this material.

COPYRIGHT © 2000
Singular Publishing Group is a division of Thomson Learning. The Thomson Learning logo is a registered trademark used herein under license

Printed in Canada
2 3 4 5 6 7 8 9 10 XXX 05 04 03 02 01 00

For more information, contact Singular Publishing Group, 401 West "A" Street, Suite 325 San Diego, CA 92101-7904; or find us on the World Wide Web at http://www.singpub.com

Library of Congress Cataloging-in-Publication Data:
ISBN: 1-565-93992-1

CONTENTS

PREFACE

The single greatest cause of preventable hearing loss is from noise exposure. Between occupational exposure and exposure to recreational noises such as music, hearing health care professionals will experience a large challenge in order to provide the optimal hearing protection program to their clients and patients. *Noise Control: A Primer* offers a well balanced review of the research and clinical literature pertaining to noise exposure. The authors represent three distinct, yet related areas, of research and clinical practiceÑthe engineer, the audiologist, and the psychophysicist.

Noise control: A Primer is written for audiologists, engineers, and industrial hygienists, and those who have an interest in noise and its effects. Chapter 1 presents an overview of the physics of sound and noise in an understandable, yet rigorous manner. Chapter 2 introduces and reviews much of what is known about the human ear and how we hear. The last twenty years has seen a tremendous revolution in our understanding of the ear and the hearing mechanism. Chapter 3 overviews both the auditory effects and the nonauditory effects of noise exposure (e.g. sleep alteration and learning), and presents a balanced review of the information and of many of the controversies about the potential effects of noise. Chapter 4 delineates the parameters and approaches to the correct measurement of noise in the industrial workplace. Chapter 5 concerns various forms of hearing protection (including both acoustic and electrical systems), along with relevant data concerning the differences between real life attenuation and laboratory studies. Chapter 6 sets forth the necessary aspects of a noise control program in order to minimize the effects of noise exposure. Chapter 7 reviews those regulations and standards concerning noise in the workplace. And finally, an extensive reference section is provided with over 160 references for further reading.

Noise Control: A Primer is meant to be used as an introductory text in courses on noise and its effects, and as an invaluable reference for those already working in the field.

Alberto Behar, B.A.Sc., P.Eng.
Marshall Chasin, M.Sc., Reg. CASLPO, Aud(C)
Margaret Cheesman, Ph.D.

Sound and Noise

This book concerns noise and sound. Everybody has some ideas on what noise and sound are, although many will have difficulty defining the difference between them. Noise and sound are basically physical phenomena (although, as we will see later, there is a definition of noise that is subjective in nature), and their properties have to be defined so that all related terms are properly used. In this chapter the basic concepts of noise and sound will be defined and explained. The mathematical support for those concepts has been basically eliminated for the purpose of simplification. In doing so, the reader will need not more than the concepts acquired in high school physics.

Sound is defined in two ways. By the definition that deals with its physical characteristics, *sound is an oscillation in pressure in an elastic medium which is capable of evoking the sensation of hearing.* Thus there must be a source of sound and also an elastic medium, such as the air, other gases, liquids, or solids. Conversely, if there is no medium, there is no sound, meaning there cannot be sound on the moon, since there is no air. Also, the oscillation in pressure must be able to cause a sensation of hearing (later in the text, it will be explained that there are certain requirements for such oscillations to elicit a hearing sensation).

By the second definition of sound, related mostly to the physiological effect from noise, *sound is the sensation of hearing excited by an acoustic oscillation.* Here, again, the two issues to be taken into account are the **acoustic oscillation** and the **sensation of hearing**. Therefore, in a way, both definitions are similar, since each refers to the physical and the physiological aspects of the sound.

There are also two definitions of **noise**. One, related to its physical properties, defines noise as *a sound, generally random in nature, the spectrum of which does not exhibit clearly defined frequency components.*

In the second more subjective definition, noise is *any unwanted sound*. The old saying equivalent to this definition is "sound is what I do, noise is what my neighbor does!"

For simplicity, in this book noise and sound will be used as synonyms.

VIBRATORY MOVEMENT AND ACOUSTICAL OSCILLATIONS

There are different types of motions. With respect to the *direction* of the motion, for example, the object (in acoustics we deal usually with something small, such as a particle or a molecule) may travel in a straight line, or it may change direction either in a determined way or at random. Then there can be differences in *speed*: sometimes the particle can travel at a constant speed, sometimes the speed can change following a certain pattern or randomly.

Finally, there is a particular type of motion, in which the particle *moves alternatively back and forth around a middle position* in the same way as a child's swing moves up and down, or as is seen in the motion of a weight suspended from an elastic band. In both cases, if left by themselves, the objects will remain in a neutral position (where they may stay forever if not disturbed). Once in motion, they oscillate around that particular, neutral position. Their speed reaches a maximum when they pass through this neutral position. The speed decreases slowly as they approach the maximum distances from the neutral position, and it becomes zero when they change the direction of the motion—for example going from up to down or from down to up.

Figure 1–1A illustrates the motion of a weight suspended from a spring and Figure 1–1B shows the type of motion known as oscillatory. In figure 1–1B, the time is displayed on the horizontal line (the abscissa) and the displacement on the vertical line (the ordinate). Another characteristic of oscillatory motion is that the particle passes through the neutral position at regular intervals of time, called "periods." This type of motion is known as oscillatory or as vibration. Many phenomena are of this nature, some of them nonmechanical (for example, electromagnetic oscillations such as light or microwaves) and others are mechanical, such as the "acoustical oscillations" and the "mechanical vibrations." Even though both acoustical oscillations and vibrations are mechanical in nature, the term "vibrations" is used mainly for low frequency oscillations such as those generated by the operations of machines, vibrations of walls, soil, etc., while "acoustical oscillations" is used for situations involving sounds.

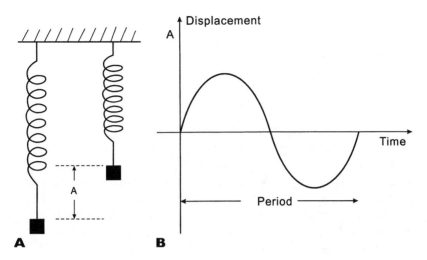

Figure 1-1. **A.** Oscillatory motion. **B.** Graph of the motion.

CHARACTERISTICS OF SOUND WAVES

Amplitude and Frequency

Like all oscillatory phenomena, sound waves are characterized by two magnitudes. One is the **amplitude**, which is the distance between the instantaneous location of the particle that is vibrating and the neutral position, where this particle remains when not in motion. The amplitude changes constantly between zero and the maximum value, as a function of the time (as shown in Figure 1–B). On many occasions, amplitude is the maximum value of the sound of interest (sometimes defined as "peak amplitude"). The amplitude corresponds to the subjective sensation of loudness: the larger the amplitude the louder the sound.

Frequency, which is the other magnitude, is defined as the number of times per second that a particle reaches the same position going in the same direction. Frequency is measured in Hertz (Hz) or in kilohertz (kHz); 1 kHz = 1000 Hz (Hertz used to be called cycles per second; cps).

The human ear can perceive sounds that have frequencies between about 20 and 20,000 Hz, depending on the hearing sensitivity of the person. Speech frequencies are mainly comprised of sounds between 500 and 5000 Hz. Some animals, such as dogs, can perceive sounds at frequencies much higher than 20,000 Hz (this is known as ultrasound). Elephants, on the other hand, perceive infrasound, that is, sounds at frequencies lower than 20 Hz.

The frequency of a sound corresponds to our sensation of pitch: the higher the frequency, the higher the pitch of the sound. For example, the hum of the refrigerator is sound comprised mainly of low frequencies, while the ringing of a telephone is a sound with its energy concentrated mainly in the high frequencies.

Pure and Complex Sounds

When a tuning fork is excited either by being hit or by electromagnetic means, its arms go into an oscillatory motion (explained previously). Since the frequency of the fork is within the limits of audition (20 to 20,000 Hz), a person in the vicinity will perceive the sound. The tuning fork, used in music, vibrates at a single frequency of 440 Hz. Consequently, the sound that it produces also has a single frequency (known as the tone of A_4). This type of sound is called "pure tone," because it contains only one frequency.

On the other hand, almost all sounds encountered in nature are the result of complex oscillations at many frequencies, and are thus called "complex sounds." In such sounds, there is often a frequency where most of the energy is concentrated (called the "fundamental frequency"), while the rest of the sound is distributed at other frequencies, that are multiples of that fundamental frequency: these are called "harmonics."

Frequency content and the distribution of its energy make one sound different from another. This particular blend helps us recognize if a sound is originated by a violin or by a human voice even when both are emitting the same tone (with the same fundamental frequency).

Figure 1–2A represents the frequency content (spectrum) of a pure tone generated by a tuning fork; Figure 1–2B shows a complex sound generated by a blower and its motor. It can clearly be seen that while all of the energy is concentrated at only one frequency in the case of the tuning fork, the energy of the blower is distributed almost over the whole spectrum.

Sound Spectrum and Frequency Bands

The graph in Figure 1–2 is the way used by scientists to represent the frequency content of a sound (or the frequency spectrum, as it is also known). The frequency is always represented in the abscissa and the sound level in the ordinate. The scale in the abscissa is always logarithmic. Therefore, the distances between the frequencies are proportional to the logarithm of the frequencies. This is why there is the same distance every time the frequency is doubled. For example, there is the same distance between the frequencies of 125 and 250 Hz as between

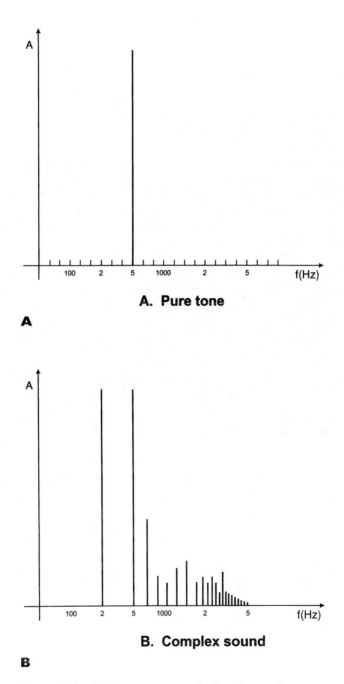

A. Pure tone

B. Complex sound

Figure 1-2. **A.** Pure tone spectrum. **B.** Complex sound spectrum.

4000 and 8000 Hz. In most cases, such as industrial noise, environmental noise, hearing conservation applications, etc., the analysis of the energy content is made only between 125 and 8000 Hz. When studying the sound properties of materials, they are measured only between 125 and 4000 Hz.

In many situations there is a need to determine energy distribution as a function of the frequency. This is, for example, the case in noise control, where the type of controls and the materials to be used will depend precisely on where the energy is concentrated.

It is impractical and time consuming to measure the energy at each frequency (e.g., at 100 Hz, 101 Hz, 102 Hz, etc.). Instead, the spectrum of the sound is "divided" into "slices" called "frequency bands."[1] The width of a frequency band depends on how detailed the analysis has to be performed. The most commonly used bands are the octave bands (1/1 bands), where the upper frequency is twice as high as the lower one. On other occasions, there is a need to determine the exact frequency at which most of the noise is concentrated (for example, when there is a distinct pure tone coming out of an exhaust stack). In this case, the analysis is done by using one-third octave bands (1/3 octave bands). There are three 1/3 octave bands in each octave band.

The octave bands as well as the third-octave bands are known by the frequency that is at the center of each band. They are all normalized internationally, so that whenever one mentions, for instance, the octave band of 1000 Hz, it is understood that this is the octave band centered at 1000 Hz.

Table 1–1 shows the frequencies of the octave and the 1/3 octave bands between 100 Hz and 10 kHz, normalized by national and international standards.

In most situations, when an octave or a 1/3 octave band analysis is performed, the result is represented graphically as a broken line that connects the centers of the bands. The spectrum of the blower in Figure 1–2B is shown again in Figure 1–3A but analyzed in octave bands and in Figure 1–3B in 1/3 octave bands.

THE MEDIUM AND SOUND PROPAGATION

It is a well known phenomenon that sound propagates (travels) away from the source: that is how a sound (speech, noise, etc.) is perceived at a distance.

In most situations, because we are immersed in an ocean of air, we speak in terms of propagation through the air. However, sound also propagates through a liquid medium: this is how somebody swimming underwater can also hear when someone is talking to him. The same applies to solid media: we can hear a conversation that is taking place in

---

[1]This is done using instruments called frequency analyzers, devices we will discuss later in the chapter on acoustical instruments.

TABLE 1-1. Normalized Frequency Bands

Frequency	Octave Bands	1/3 Octave Bands
100		X
125	X	X
160		X
200		X
250	X	X
315		X
400		X
500	X	X
630		X
800		X
1000	X	X
1250		X
1600		X
2000	X	X
2500		X
3150		X
4000	X	X
5000		X
6300		X
8000	X	X
10000		X

an adjacent room. When the sound waves impinge the wall between both rooms, they vibrate (obviously, this is a very minuscule vibration), transmitting the sound to the other room.

Sound propagates through the air by so-called pressure waves. In our previous example of the tuning fork, the motion is transmitted to the molecules that surround the fork's arms so that they in turn start oscillating. The molecules in turn "push" one another in the direction of the propagation of the sound. Therefore, at any one point in space, there will be a minuscule compression followed by a rarefaction due to the air movement, as shown in Figure 1–4. This compression is known as "sound pressure." We will be talking more on that subject further in this chapter.

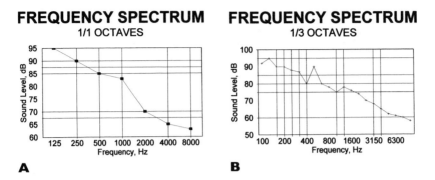

Figure I–3. A. Octave band spectrum. **B.** 1/3 octave band spectrum.

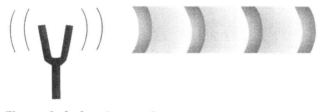

Figure I–4. Sound propagation.

SPEED OF SOUND

The speed at which the sound travels depends on the physical properties of the media it is travelling through. In general, the denser the medium, the faster the sound travels.

Table 1–2 shows the speed (in meters per second) in some typical media.

PROPAGATION PHENOMENA

When a sound source (e.g., a bell, a loudspeaker, a person talking) emits a sound, this sound disturbance travels in spherical waves around the source in a motion similar to the waves observed when a stone is thrown into the middle of a lake. The direction of propagation is defined as a straight line, perpendicular to the wave itself. The surface connecting all points undergoing the same disturbance at the same time is called the "wave front." Close to the source, the wave front is spherical and the waves are called "spherical waves." However, far away from the source,

TABLE 1-2. Speed of Sound in Selected Media

Media	Speed (m/s)
Air	332
Water	1,500
Steel	5,365

the wave's front is an almost straight line and the waves are called "plane waves."

When sound travels in the same medium its direction follows a straight line. However, when it reaches a medium of different physical characteristics, such as when going from air to water, or hitting a wall, the direction changes and several phenomena occur that will be examined in the following sections.

Reflection

Reflection is one of the phenomena observed when the sound that is travelling in one medium reaches another medium. Figure 1–5 illustrates this situation, where a plane sound wave reaches a wall (a medium different from the air the wave is travelling through) and it is partially reflected. The energy of the sound in the first medium will increase because of the contribution of the reflected sound and will become louder. As a matter of fact, every time the sound reaches a wall, the reflection increases its amplitude, in the same way a mirror can increase the light from a lamp. Reflections from the walls and ceiling make it easier for an actor to be heard in a theater that is enclosed than in an open one. By the same effect, if a machine is located close to a wall, the noise from the machine will increase, because of the reflected sound energy.

A particular effect from reflection is the echo. This is the phenomenon by which, when clapping hands in proximity to a large wall, a hill, a forest, etc., we perceive a second sound that is repeat of the original. To be perceived as an echo, the time delay between the direct and the reflected sound has to be longer than 1/10 of a second.[2] If this is not the case, we perceive the sound as "enlarged" in duration. The result (the sound perceived as longer) is what is known as reverberation; that is, the result of multiple reflections with time delays shorter than 0.1 second.

[2]This is the length of time our brain needs to process the second, reflected sound as distinct from the direct one.

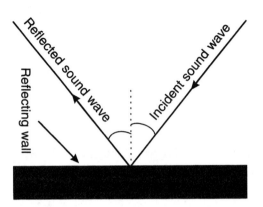

Figure 1-5. Sound reflection.

Refraction

Refraction is another phenomenon that occurs when the advancing sound wave impinges upon another medium. As explained above, at the interface between both media part of the energy is reflected. The remaining energy penetrates the second medium. This energy is known as "refracted" and the phenomenon as "refraction." Figure 1–6 illustrates a situation when the incident wave reaches the surface of a lake. Part of the energy from the incident wave is reflected by the water back into the air. The rest is refracted into the water. This phenomenon, very common in real life, allows for the transmission of the sound into a second medium. It is governed by certain rules regarding the direction and the amplitude of the refracted waves, rules that we will not examine further in this chapter.

Diffraction

When dealing with light (another vibratory phenomenon), it is a common experience to create a shadow by interposing a non-transparent object in front of a light source. Because the light *does* not bend around the corners, we create a shadow. This is not the case with sound, where the sound does "bend" around the corners. This is how the honking from a car horn is clearly perceived even if the car itself is not visible. Diffraction is the phenomenon observed when sound waves reach a dis-

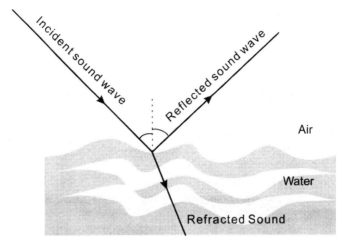

Figure 1–6. Sound refraction.

continuity (such as the edge of a barrier or an opening in a wall) in a different medium. The discontinuity generates a sound wave with the same characteristics as the incident wave. Figures 1–7A and 1–7B illustrate this phenomenon.

Because of the diffraction phenomenon, the sound barriers often erected on the sides of highways do not completely protect the homes behind them and the traffic sound is "spilled" over the barriers, even though attenuated.

Interference

When sound waves travelling in one direction are reflected and return to the original medium, the air molecules are subjected to two motions: one from the incident wave (the one originated from the source) and one from the reflected wave. This phenomenon is called "interference." Depending on the amplitudes of both waves, it may happen that the resulting motion is zero, meaning that the sound has been eliminated. This principle has been progressively exploited for the so-called "active noise control" used in noise control devices and hearing protectors.

Free Field

When a source of noise (e.g., a speaker, a machine) is located in the open, far from reflective surfaces (for example, in a football field), the sound

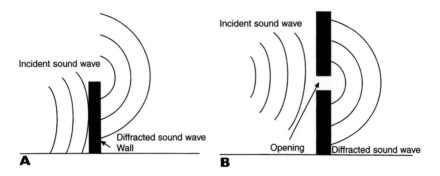

Figure 1-7. Sound diffraction. **A.** On an edge. **B.** Through a hole.

waves propagate freely until they reach some obstacle. They are then reflected and some of their energy is returned toward the source. Depending on the characteristics of the reflecting walls, the reflected energy may be so small that its importance is negligible. Free field, or free field propagation, is by definition a situation where the reflected energy is much smaller than the incident one. In that case, as the distance between the source and the receiver increases, the amplitude of the sound is reduced, and it is perceived each time fainter and fainter until at a certain distance it is no longer perceptible.

Reverberant Field

In an enclosed space, the sound energy travels from the source to the limiting surfaces (floor, ceiling, walls), bounces off them, and then returns to the origin. If the limiting surfaces are highly reflective there will be no reduction of the sound energy within the enclosure because of the multiple reflections and the amplitude of the sound will remain approximately constant everywhere, independently of the location where the sound is generated. As a consequence, even after the source has been turned off, the sound reverberates for a long time. This is particularly noticeable in warehouses, churches, caves, etc., with acoustically hard surfaces (such as walls, floor and ceilings without acoustic treatment). A sound of short duration emitted in a reverberant field persists for a long time before its energy has been depleted by absorption through the air and by transmission through the walls. The harder the limiting surfaces, the longer the sound persists.

The effect of the reverberation on speech intelligibility is very important. Speech is a complex combination of vowels and consonants which have to be clearly separated in time. The effect of reverberation is to blend them all together, so that before the amplitude of a syllable has decreased, the following syllable is already coming up and has a similar amplitude. The net effect is that intelligibility is greatly reduced, and unless the speaker is close to the listener the latter will have difficulties in understanding what has been said.

The same phenomenon happens with music. To be clearly perceived, the reverberation has to be kept within limits. This is why the first thing to be controlled during the design of a theater and/or music hall is the reverberation.

ACOUSTIC MAGNITUDES

Sound Pressure

The weight of the air that surrounds the planet Earth puts a pressure on its surface that at sea level is equal to:

$$1 \text{ atmosphere} = 101,325 \text{ pascals (Pa)} = 101,325 \text{ newtons/m}^2$$

The nature of the atmospheric pressure is such that its value is almost constant, with slight variations due to the weather conditions that occur over relatively long periods of time.

Sound pressure, as we know it, consists of alternative variations of the pressure that occur with a frequency between 20 Hz and 20 kHz. The magnitude of this pressure is extremely small. For instance, the minimum pressure that can elicit the sensation of our hearing at 1000 Hz is in the order of 0.000020 pascal or 20 micropascals. The so-called threshold of pain, that is, a sound capable of hurting our ears, is only about 20 Pa, almost 5,000 times smaller than the atmospheric pressure.

Sound Power

Sound power, that is, the rate at which sound energy is emitted, is also very small. It is expressed usually in watts and picowatts (1 picowatt = 10^{-12} watt). Sound power is seldom used in most practical applications.

Sound Intensity

Sound intensity is the flow of sound power through the unity of surface area. Lately, the use of the sound intensity measurements and applications has become more popular, because of the development of specialized instrumentation capable of measuring this type of magnitude. Its use is limited mainly to noise control applications, since it allows for determining which part of the surface of a noise source is responsible for a particular noise emission. The applications are limited to large noise sources and, mainly, during the design process of the source.

The term "sound intensity" is often used as a synonym for sound level, as in the expression "the intensity of the sound is [so many] decibels." Obviously, sound intensity and sound level are two completely different concepts and should not be used as synonyms.

LEVELS AND DECIBELS

Definitions

Human hearing deals with a very extensive range of sound pressures—of the order of 1,000,000 times between the threshold of hearing and the threshold of pain. One very convenient way of "compressing" such a wide range is by using a logarithmic scale. Then, instead of the sound pressure per se, we deal in terms of sound pressure levels, that are proportional to the logarithm of the sound pressure.

The mathematical expression of the levels, in terms of decibels (dB) is:

$$\text{Level (dB)} = 10 \log (\text{magnitude}/\text{reference})$$

where the magnitude is the sound pressure and the reference sound pressure is 20 micropascal.

In this book we limit ourselves to sound pressure levels measured in dB, although the sound power as well as the sound intensity can also be expressed as sound power level and sound intensity level.

Table 1–3 compares the sound levels and the sound pressures corresponding to some commonly found situations/sources.

TABLE 1–3. Sound Levels and Sound Pressure Levels

Situation	Sound Pressure Level (dB)	Sound Pressure (micropascals)
Threshold of pain	120	20,000,000
Discotheque	110	6,500,000
Textile mill	90	650,000
Office environment	60	20,000
Soft whisper at 2 meters	35	1,000
Threshold of hearing	0	20

Combining Levels

When two sources are operating simultaneously, the resulting level is not the arithmetic sum of both individual levels. Because we are dealing with logarithmic magnitudes, the addition is done in a different way. Without getting into too many details, for our purposes it is sufficient to remember the following two rules that apply to most situations found in real life:

(a) **The sum of two equal levels is equal to one of them plus 3 dB.**
Examples: 90 dB + 90 dB = 93 dB
45 dB + 45 dB = 48 dB

(b) **The sum of two levels, one of which is 9 or more dB lower than the second, is equal to the highest level.**
Examples: 90 dB + 80 dB = 90 dB
45 dB + 36 dB = 45 dB

For the purpose of calculating the sound level resulting from the sum of two sound levels, Table 1–4 "Sum of Sound Levels" shows the number of dB that have to be added to the higher of two levels.

Example: Adding 57 dB and 59 dB: their difference is 59 − 57 = 2 dB. Therefore 2 dB should be added to the higher level (59 dB), resulting in an overall level of 61 dB.

The above example can be used to prove that when there are several noise sources in one room (several machines, printers, etc), the overall level depends mainly on the noisiest of all. Therefore, there is no

TABLE 1–4. Sum of Sound Levels

Difference Between the Two Levels	dB to Be Added to the Highest Level
9	0.
7	1.4
6	1.0
4	1.5
2	2.1
1	2.5
0	3.0

point in silencing some of the noise sources, unless the noisiest is treated first. Also, silencing a source with a sound level 9 dB lower than another will not have a noticeable effect on the overall noise level.

WEIGHTING NETWORKS: A, B, AND C

The human ear does not perceive sounds of the same pressure but different frequencies as equally loud. It is most sensitive at the frequencies between 500 and 5000 Hz, which correspond loosely to the frequencies of human speech. Also, human hearing is not damaged equally by sounds at different frequencies. It just happens that sounds at frequencies within the most sensitive range are also the most damaging.

The above properties of the ear offer an attractive way of measuring noise for the purpose of assessing the risk of hearing loss from excessive noise. All devices that measure sound levels ("sound level meters"; abbreviated "SLMs") are equipped with an electronic filter that simulates the perception of how loud the noise is as well as its potential risk for hearing. This filter is known as "A" filter, or A-frequency weighting filter.[3] Whenever a sound is measured using this filter, results are expressed as dBA. All national and international standards, as well as all state, provincial and municipal regulations that deal with environmental noise and hearing loss, require that noise levels be measured in dBA.

There is another filter used for hearing conservation purposes (see Figure 1–8). It is known as the "C" filter. When a hearing protector is to be used, it is necessary to calculate the noise level under the protector (i.e., the noise level reaching the protected ear). To do so, the attenuation of the hearing protector, expressed in NRR[4] is subtracted from the ambient noise level measured using the C-weighting filter. (For more details see the chapter on Hearing Protectors.)

Some SLMs have also a "B" filter, that was used in the past but which has no practical use at the present time.

NOISE EXPOSURE LEVEL

Hearing loss results from exposure to loud noise for long periods of time —months and years (except in cases of accidental exposure to very high

---

[3]The A-frequency weighting approximates the ear's response characteristics for low level sound, below about 55 dB. B-frequency weighting approximates the frequency response of the ear between 55 and 85 dB. Finally, C-weighting corresponds to the frequency response for sound levels higher than 85 dB.

[4]NRR: Noise Reduction Rating, in dB, is an expression for the attenuation provided by a hearing protector.

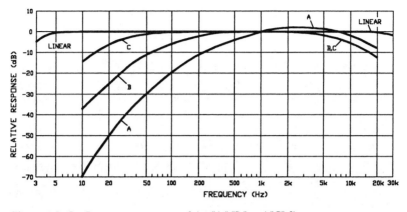

Figure I-8. Frequency response of the "A," "B," and "C" filters.

level impulse noise or air blasts). Therefore, in addition to determining the instantaneous sound level, it is necessary to obtain information about the total sound energy that is entering the ear when assessing if this noise presents a risk to the noise exposed person.

In this case, the magnitude that is measured is the **noise exposure level**—that is, the average noise level a person is exposed to during a certain period of time. The mathematical expression is:

$$L_{ex,T} = 10 \log 1/T\Sigma t_i 10^{0.1L_i}$$

where $L_{ex,T}$ is the noise exposure level, during the time T

L_i are the individual sound levels measured at the intervals i of time,

t_i is the total duration of each measurement, and

T is the normalized duration of the work day (or week).

When the measurement is performed during the entire period of work, the noise exposure level is known as "equivalent noise level," abbreviated as L_{eq} and its expression becomes

$$L_{eq} = 10 \log \Sigma 10^{0.1L_i}$$

The noise exposure level is measured using a noise dosimeter, as will be seen in Chapter 4, Noise Measurements.

CONTINUOUS, INTERRUPTED, AND IMPULSE NOISES

As the name indicates, continuous noise is characterized by having almost no interruptions. Although the frequency content, sound level or both may change, there is no interruption of the energy flow. Examples are traffic noise from a highway, noise from a power plant, or noise from the fan of an air conditioner.

Most noises are **interrupted**, meaning that their duration is not permanent. Examples are human speech, the operation of most handheld tools, vacuum cleaners, etc.

Finally, there is **impulse noise**, such as hammer blows or gunfire, consisting of impulses of very short duration, each impulse separated from the other by periods of time that make them quite distinctive. Although there is no definition of impulse noise, most acousticians agree that impulses should be shorter than 0.5 second and be separated by a time interval of at least 0.5 second. The effect on the hearing of people exposed to impulse noise is not yet fully understood. Of the many characteristics of the impulse noise, the most damaging is the *peak level*, which is defined as the maximum instantaneous level achieved by the sound pressure level.

2

Hearing and Hearing Loss

This chapter is not intended to provide an in–depth analysis of the physics of noise and psychophysics of hearing; rather it addresses the salient features and phenomena in a nonmathematical but consistent manner. A physiological basis is provided to answer many of the typical questions that may be posed, as well as to provide a framework in order to understand the results of research.

THE HUMAN EAR

The ear is composed of several sections: the outer ear, the middle ear, and the inner ear, as well as related neurological pathways. Figure 2–1 shows the relevant anatomical features important for some of the observed characteristics of hearing. These characteristics will be discussed further.

The Outer Ear

The outer ear, the section bounded by the pinna on the lateral side and the tympanic membrane on the medial side, has two primary functions. They are an amplification of higher frequency energy (the "pinna effect") and the creation of a resonance in the 3000 Hz region that further amplifies higher frequency energy.

The pinna effect creates a high-frequency boost of sound energy above 2500 Hz, which gradually increases with frequency up to about 8 to 10 decibels (dB). The physics of this effect are simple and relate to the shorter high-frequency wavelengths reflecting from the pinna back to the opening of the ear canal. In contrast, the lower frequency energy

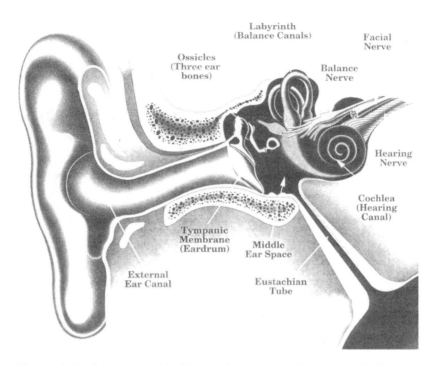

Figure 2–1. Schematic model of the ear showing some relevant anatomical features. (Courtesy of Starkey-Canada.)

range, which has longer wavelengths, is not affected by the presence of the pinna and, therefore, is not reflected back to the ear canal entrance. The "frequency-specific reflective" characteristics of sounds were described in greater detail in Chapter 1. Figure 2–2 shows this net high-frequency boost due to the presence of the pinna, as well as the ear canal resonance. The total effect is also shown.

The 3000 Hz resonance (shown in Figure 2–2) is inversely related to the length of the ear canal and corresponds to a quarter-wavelength resonance. For people with very long ear canals, this resonance that is typically 15 to 20 dB tends to be at a slightly lower frequency than that of "short-eared" individuals. A wavelength resonance can be heard when blowing across the top of a length of pipe; the longer the pipe, the lower the resonant frequency. High-frequency fundamental or harmonic energy is enhanced in intensity because of these two properties of the outer ear.

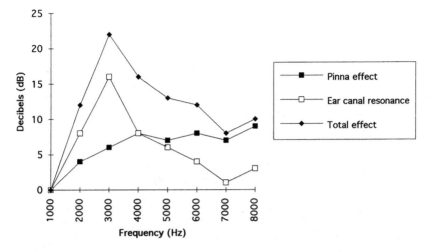

Figure 2–2. The physical structure of the outer ear yields a high-frequency boost. The two elements of this boost are related to the pinna effect and the ear canal resonance.

The Middle Ear

The middle ear has three major characteristics that relate to the acoustics of the sound that a person ultimately receives: *impedance matching, temporary reduction of high-intensity sounds,* and *pressure release.*

Impedance Matching

Why do we have a middle ear? The primary reason is to match the characteristics of the air in the ear canal to that of the fluid in the inner ear. The middle ear can be thought of as a transformer for a train set. When we play with an electric train set we must be cautious to ensure that the 120 volts coming from the electric socket in the wall is stepped down to match the 10 to 12 volt requirements of the train set. Subsequently, all train sets come with a matching transformer (or simply a transformer) that electronically matches the wall power supply to the needs of the train set. This is known as *impedance matching*.

Similarly, the middle ear serves to match the mechanical characteristics of sound in the air to that of the fluid in the inner ear. Approximately 99% of the energy is lost when sounds go through an air–fluid barrier. This converts to 30 dB (i.e., $10 \times \log 10^{-3}$, for those who like logarithms) and can be noticed when swimming under the water while listening to someone above the surface. If there was no middle ear, our hearing sensitivity would be reduced by about 30 dB. However, as observed in Figure 2–3, the mid-frequency sensitivity is improved dramatically because of the middle ear. The effects of the middle ear are less beneficial for very low- and very high-frequency sounds.

Figure 2–3 (from Rosowski, 1991) shows a calculated middle ear efficiency for three species: human, chinchilla, and cat. Note how the human middle ear efficiency falls off above 1000 Hz. Because the human middle ear is so inefficient for high-frequency sounds, a middle ear pathology generally does not affect the high-frequency sound transmission.

Temporary Reduction of High-intensity Sounds

The middle ear also provides for a temporary reduction of high–intensity sounds. This is related to a small muscle that is connected to the stapes bone in the middle ear, called the stapedius muscle. Such a muscle, which contracts with high-intensity sound (the *stapedial reflex*), serves to lessen the intensity of the person's own voice, especially for the mid- and low-frequency sounds (Zakrisson, Borg, Liden, & Nilsson, 1980; Borg, Counter, & Rossler, 1984; Borg & Counter, 1989; Borg,

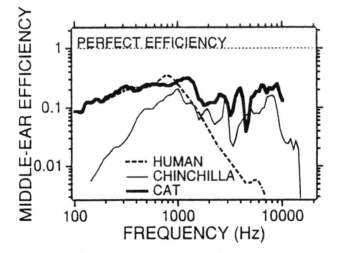

Figure 2–3. Improved mid-frequency sensitivity because of the physical structure of the middle ear. Calculated improved middle ear efficiencies from three species—human, chinchilla, and the cat. (Reprinted with permission from Rosowski, J. [1991]. "The effects of external- and middle-ear filtering on auditory threshold and noise-induced hearing loss." *Journal of the Acoustical Society of America, 90,* 124–135. Copyright 1991 Acoustical Society of America.)

Canlon, & Engström, 1995). However, such a neurological reflex adapts or gradually loses its function over 15 to 20 seconds. Therefore, eliciting this reflex prior to a sound such as a loud noise impulse (by humming) may serve to lessen the damaging effects, but the duration of the effect will not be long lasting.

An upper limit for the protection from temporary threshold shift of the stapedius reflex can be greater than 20 dB in birds (Borg & Counter, 1989), and 15 dB in humans with malfunctioning stapedial reflexes due to Bell's palsy (Zakrisson et al., 1980). Borg, Nilsson, & Counter (1983) also noted a permanent threshold shift in excess of 30 dB in rabbits with a surgically de-innervated stapedius muscle. Possibly the most important factor to explain why some individuals are more susceptible to hearing loss from noise exposure than others is because the latter have a stapedial reflex that becomes activated at a lower intensity level, thus providing a greater amount of protection (Borg, Canlon, & Engström, 1995).

Pressure Release

A third feature of the middle ear is pressure release. A trapped volume of air such as that found in the middle ear would not be able to respond to changes in environmental air pressure unless a "pressure valve" was utilized. The eustachian tube serves such a function. Typically, this tube is closed and is surrounded by mucous membrane. When a person yawns or swallows, the tube opens, allowing the air pressure to equalize between the environment and the middle ear. When a person has a cold, swelling occurs in the mucous membrane, thus clamping shut the eustachian tube. Pressure equalization is therefore very difficult during such a time and a temporary mild hearing loss may occur.

However, this pressure release can work both ways. Not only can the middle ear pressure be equalized with the environment, but positive middle ear pressure relative to the environment can be established by extreme effort during lifting. Forceful subglottal pressure, such as that necessary to lift heavy objects, can cause air to be forced up through the eustachian tube into the middle ear space (the "Valsalva maneuver"). Such a pressure differential can cause a slight temporary hearing loss that can actually benefit the worker by acting as a mild earplug (Chasin, 1989).

Problems with the outer or middle ear (such as ear wax buildup, tympanic membrane perforation, middle ear infection, or a stiffening of the middle ear ossicles or bones) lead to *conductive hearing losses*. With a few exceptions, conductive hearing losses are medically treatable. Hearing loss related to the inner ear and associated neurological structures is referred to as a *sensorineural hearing loss* and, with a very few exceptions, is not medically treatable.

The Inner Ear

The inner ear (or cochlea) is a fluid-filled, snail-shaped structure about the size of the small fingernail. Running the length of the cochlea over the full two-and-one-half spiral turns is a thin sheet called the *basilar membrane*. Sitting upon this membrane is the *organ of Corti* that contains approximately 15,500 nerve endings or hair cells (Spoendlin, 1986). The structure of sound transduction in the cochlea is similar to that of a piano keyboard: low-frequency sounds are transduced on one end while the higher frequency sounds are transduced from the other end. Specifically, in the cochlea, high-frequency sounds are transduced by those hair cells nearer to the stapes footplate of the middle ear, while those that transduce the lower-frequency sounds are found in the inner-most turns of this snail-shaped organ. There is approximately a one octave change every 1.25 mm along the basilar membrane (about 30 mm in length in adults) in the cochlea.

One quarter (about 3500) of the nerve fibers are inner hair cells and three quarters (about 12,000) are outer hair cells (Spoendlin, 1986). Approximately 90 to 95% of inner hair cells are associated with sensory or *afferent* (toward the brain) neurons, whereas only 5 to 10% of the outer hair cells have afferent innervation. The outer hair cells are mostly innervated by motor or *efferent* (away from the brain) neurons. The cochlea presents us with a startling irregularity—the majority of the hair cells are innervated by efferent neurons, not afferent.

Up until the late 1970s, the physiology of these common efferent nerve fibers was not understood, but recent research indicates that they function as a feedback loop modulating the function of the inner ear. Figure 2–4 illustrates the efferent-induced feedback change. However, other researchers have shown that this feedback loop in the cochlea has its greatest effect for lower intensity sounds. Specifically, "the outer hair cells are mostly motor rather than sensory units, amplifying the motion of faint sounds below 60 dB SPL (sound pressure level) and somehow stimulating the inner hair cells" (Berlin, 1994). These hair cells gradually lose their amplifying function for more intense sounds, with the result that while they improve the sensitivity for quiet sounds, they have no appreciable affect for more intense sounds. In this sense, outer hair cells function as a level-dependent filter.

Most people with normal hearing have emissions emanating from the outer hair cells in the inner ear. These "otoacoustic emissions" can be measured in the outer ear canal and have been used as indicators of hearing function (Lonsbury-Martin, Harris, Hawkins, Stagner, & Martin, 1990). Specifically, otoacoustic emissions are measurable in individuals with normal outer and middle ears as long as there is less than about a 30 dB sensorineural hearing loss. Although there is a large

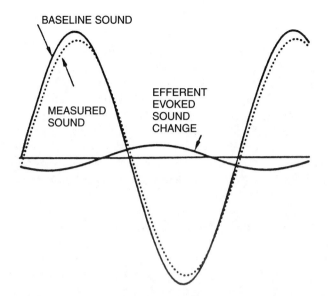

Figure 2-4. Schematic of an efferent (outgoing) nerve-induced feedback change to the outer hair cells. (Reprinted with permission from Guinan, J. J. [1986]. Effect of efferent neural activity on cochlear mechanics." In G. Cianfrone & F. Grandori [Eds.], *Cochlear mechanics and otoacoustic emissions* (pp. 53–62). [*Scandinavian Audiology*, Suppl. 25] Copyright 1986 Scandinavian Audiology.)

degree of variability with such measurements, recent research has indicated improved reliability utilizing otoacoustic emission delay measurements (Mahoney & Kemp, 1995).

An interesting finding is that hearing damage occurs to the outer hair cells prior to inner hair cell damage. Therefore, an abnormal otoacoustic emission test result may be observed before a measureable hearing loss is detected utilizing conventional pure-tone hearing testing. It is not clear why outer hair cells are more prone to damage than inner hair cells. One possible reason may be related to the physical location of the hair cells in the cochlea. The inner hair cells sit at the edge of a bony shelf (osseous spiral lamina) in the cochlea so they are not as affected by the motion of the basilar membrane as are the outer hair cells, which sit directly on this moving base (Lim, 1986). It is possible that this constant movement (and constant shearing by the tectorial membrane situated above the hair cells) eventually causes the outer hair cells to lose their transducing properties before the inner hair cells do.

As discussed above, the inner ear has a complicated neurological structure associated with it that includes feedback loops. In addition to this structure is the auditory cortex where much of auditory cognition occurs. It is this central area that is related to an individual's ability to be able to attribute pitch to a sound. Approximately one person in 1500 can perform this task with amazing accuracy (called perfect or absolute pitch) and this is thought to be related to the organization of the central structures (Bachem, 1955). People with perfect pitch generally maintain this ability despite significant cochlear damage (Langendorf, 1992). Recent evidence suggests that this is also the site of many forms of tinnitus which will be discussed in more detail later in this chapter.

THE SHAPE OF THINGS TO COME

Hearing losses from a wide range of noise sources have similar audiometric patterns. The low-frequency sensitivity is either normal or near normal, whereas sensitivity in the 3000 to 6000 Hz region is reduced. Yet, the acuity of an individual to an 8000 Hz sound is much better and like the lower frequencies can be normal or near normal. This *audiometric notch*, shown in Figure 2–5, is characteristic of many forms of damage from noise exposure.

Audiometric Notch

What are the causes of the nonmonotonic nature of noise-induced hearing loss that creates an audiometric notch? Several explanations have been proposed for this notch. These include (a) a poor blood supply to the part of the cochlea that corresponds to the 3000 to 6000 Hz region (Crow, Guild, & Polvogot, 1934); (b) a greater susceptibility for damage of the supporting structures of the hair cells in this region (Bohne, 1976); (c) the orientation of the stapes footplate into the inner ear is such that its primary force vector aims toward those hair cells in this region, with the effect of eventual failure because of the constant hydromechanical action (Hilding, 1953; Schuknecht & Tonndorf, 1960); and (d) permanent noise exposure has its greatest effect approximately one-half octave above the peak frequency of the noise spectrum. Since all spectra are enhanced at 3000 Hz by the outer ear canal resonance, the greatest loss will be in the 4000 to 6000 Hz region (Tonndorf, 1976; Caiazzo & Tonndorf, 1977). Because of these phenomena, hearing losses due to noise (including music) exposure are relatively easy to spot.

However, many clinical cases of music or noise exposure do not possess an audiometric notch. Indeed, Barrs, Althoff, Krueger, and

AUDIOGRAM
Frequency in Hertz

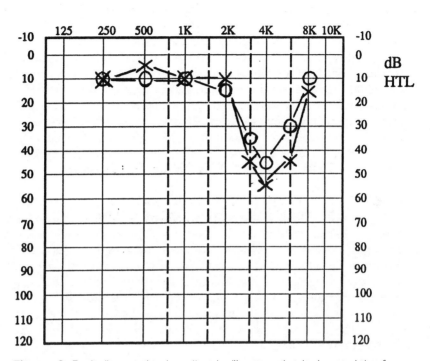

Figure 2-5. Audiogram showing a "notched" pattern that is characteristic of many forms of noise (and music) exposure.

Olsson (1994) found that only 37% of workers suffering from noise exposure possessed an audiometric notch. It is quite possible that in advanced cases of exposure or advanced age where there is a significant age-related hearing loss ("presbycusis"), the hearing sensitivity at 8000 Hz may have also deteriorated, leaving a flat audiometric configuration. In addition, depending on the noise spectrum, the frequency region of greatest damage may be above the audiometric test frequencies. For example, using data derived from violin players, the frequency of greatest damage can be at 8000 Hz, and unless a higher frequency pure tone were to be assessed (e.g. 10,000 Hz), a notch would not be apparent.

Alberti (1982) argued that industrial noise exposure tends to be symmetrical. This rationale is based on the highly reverberant environment many workers find themselves in. A damaging sound from a worker's left side may be just as intense at the worker's right side, given a sufficiently reverberant environment. However, in less reverberant environments (or ones with sufficient high-frequency energy), the exposure to one ear may be significantly different than that to the contralateral ear ("head shadow"), thus resulting in an asymmetrical audiometric pattern.

Chasin (1991) studied the audiometric pattern of 68 riveters by using hand-held devices: 64 of them had audiometric asymmetries. It was found that in 88% of the 64 cases, the side of the greatest audiometric loss was opposite that of the dominant hand of the worker. That is, a right-handed riveter braced the rivet gun on their right side using their left hand as support (much like a shotgun), and their left ear was consequently much closer to the noise source. This difference in proximity of ear to the noise source accounted for the differing exposures between the two ears.

EQUAL LOUDNESS CONTOURS

Because of the acoustic characteristics of the outer ear, the "matching transformer" characteristics of the middle ear, and the sensitivity and neurological integration of the inner ear, the relationship between the intensities of sound at various frequencies can be complicated.

Figure 2–6 shows part of this information—the least intense sound that a person can hear across the frequency range. This curve can be thought of as an *equal loudness contour*. That is, this is a curve where all frequencies are judged to be equally loud. It typically takes an intense low-frequency sound just to be audible, and a much less intense mid-frequency sound just to be audible.

However, do all equal loudness contours have a similar bowl shape? If we were to perform an experiment where we attempted to obtain judgments on the similarities of the loudness of many tones, we would ultimately come up with a full range of contours—equally loud judgments of different frequencies. Clinically, this is not done because of time constraints, the amount of training required by the listener, and the degree of variability in the data. However, data are available from many experiments that show similar results: equal loudness contours tend to "flatten out" as the test intensity is increased.

Figure 2–7 shows this feature of flattening out. The bottom curve (threshold of normal hearing under earphones is very bowl shaped (identical to that found in Figure 2–6), but the bowl becomes a flattened dish at a test level of 60 dB and above. These curves have also been named after the various researchers who have studied them. The most popular alias is the *Fletcher-Munson curve* after Fletcher & Munson (1933), but similar data have also been obtained by Sivan & White

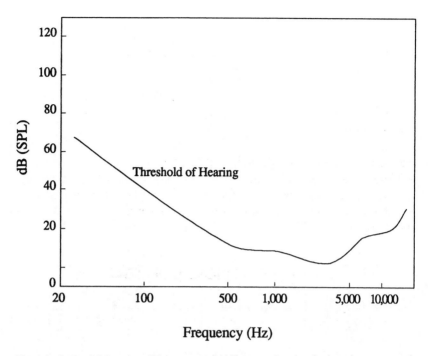

Figure 2–6. Minimum audible pressure (MAP) curve showing the least intense sounds (i.e., the thresholds) of a normal hearing person, across frequency. Note an increased sensitivity for the mid-frequencies.

(1933), and Stevens (1961), to name but a few. There are subtle differences and they probably relate to testing technique, equipment setup, and subject variability. Exact values for equal loudness contours should thus be viewed with caution.

When hearing is tested on an audiometer, data similar to the bottom curve are used to calibrate the test machine. A reading of 0 dB HL ("hearing Level" or HL) on the audiometer could represent a wide range of sound pressure levels depending on the test frequency. A flat "audiogram" at 0 dB HL, which is a graphic measure of hearing, would indicate normal hearing. A 30 dB loss in the hearing at 6000 Hz (an audiometric notch), which is frequently observed in the hearing of industrial workers and musicians, implies that that individual's equal loudness contour would require a 30 dB more intense level at 6000 Hz than that of a person with normal hearing. Yet if measured at a higher stimulus level, the person's equal loudness contours would tend to flatten out. This is one reason why individuals do not necessarily notice a mild hearing loss as long as people with whom they interact speak at an intense enough level.

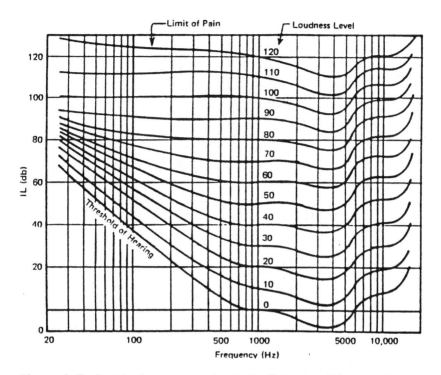

Figure 2-7. Equal loudness contours showing the "flattening out" feature as stimulus level is increased. The lowest "contour" is the threshold curve shown in Figure 2–6. (Reprinted with permission from Fletcher, H. & Munson, W. A. [1933]. "Loudness, its definition, measurement, and calculation." *Journal of the Acoustical Society of America,* 5(1), 82–108. Copyright 1933 Acoustical Society of America.)

In some sense, the typical audiogram that measures an equal loudness contour at the threshold of hearing can be thought of as an artifact. A mild loss may be viewed as completely normal if a similar equal loudness contour was instead performed at a higher level—one that would have a flattened dish shape. Only two equal loudness contours can be clinically assessed without additional training while still maintaining a high level of reliability: the *minimal audibility threshold* and the *pain threshold*. However, a person may have a very significant hearing loss and still have a normal pain threshold, so such an alternative audiogram would be rather insensitive (as well as uncomfortable). In this sense, an audiogram with a mild notch should be thought of as an early warning indicator of pathological equal loudness contours and not as the end of one's ability to communicate well in noise.

A further extension of this reasoning is that otoacoustic emission testing can be thought of as a very early warning indicator, and if our clinical function is to warn our patients of any impending damage, then otoacoustic emission testing should be part of the audiometric battery. Indeed, Martin, Champlin, and Chambers (1998) found in a recent survey of audiometric practices for 500 audiologists that 33% use otoacoustic emission testing.

UPWARD SPREAD OF MASKING

Upward spread of masking refers to the phenomenon where low-frequency sounds can not only mask out signals of the same frequency, but also can mask out some of the higher frequency signals. A low-frequency background noise masking out many of the higher frequency consonant sounds responsible for communication is a common example of this phenomenon.

Upward spread of masking was first studied in detail in the 1950s by Hirsh and Bowman (1953); Bilger and Hirsh (1956); Pickett (1959); and Jerger, Tillman, and Peterson (1960). It has extensively been studied since and appears to be related to the asymmetrical behavior of the tuning curves of the inner ear hair cells that transduce sound up to the brain. A particular hair cell that is tuned to 1000 Hz as an example, will not only respond to a 1000 Hz signal, but also to a lower frequency signal. It will not however, respond to a higher frequency signal unless that signal is very intense. Low-frequency noise energy tends to mask the higher-frequency consonants, thus limiting communication in noisy environments.

Upward spread of masking is found in varying amounts with normal hearing people, and to a greater extent with those with sensorineural hearing loss. This type of masking accounts for why some people with sensorineural hearing loss have difficulty communicating in a noisy environment, even with the assistance of amplification.

TINNITUS

Tinnitus is defined as a perceived acoustic sensation that occurs in the absence of an external sound source. It may be classified as objective or subjective. Objective tinnitus is extremely rare and can actually be audible by another person in the room. This is usually related to a vascular or muscular etiology. In contrast, subjective tinnitus is heard only by the patient.

Depending on the study, up to 30% of the population may suffer from tinnitus (Coles, 1987) and 1% of patients report that it significantly interferes with daily living (Tyler, Aran, & Dauman, 1992).

Most of the research in this area pertains to developing treatment models rather than to determining the etiology (Knox, 1993; Levine, 1994) and this is understandable given the wide range of possible site of lesions covered by the one term "tinnitus." Nevetheless, there has been some progress in the development of an animal model by Pawel Jastreboff and Jonathan Hazell (Jastreboff & Hazell, 1993; Hazell, Jastreboff, Meerton, & Conway, 1993) based not only on damage to the outer and inner hair cells, but to higher neurological structures as well. Indeed, many researchers now agree that tinnitus is localized in the auditory cortex and that this has been caused by altered input from the periphery caused by cochlear damage. That is, a sensorineural hearing loss restricts input to the brain and tinnitus is perceived. Appropriate retraining of the brain can therefore reduce the perceived tinnitus.

Other treatments for tinnitus have also appeared in the literature, such as intravenous use of lidocaine (Murai, Tyler, Harker, & Stouffer, 1992), various antidepressants (Johnson, Brummet, & Schleuning, 1993), and behavior modification and psychotherapy intervention. The use of hearing aids has been shown to reduce the annoyance of tinnitus in many subjects, as has the use of tinnitus maskers in a lesser number of subjects.

Although the approach of Jastreboff and Hazell looks quite promising, it should be pointed out that no single approach can be considered a cure. An eclectic approach that includes elements of masking, biofeedback, and psychological counseling, as well as various suppression techniques, may be the optimal clinical approach.

3

Auditory and Nonauditory Effects of Noise

This chapter provides an overview of the factors known to cause occupational hearing loss (auditory) and of the factors known to cause nonauditory effects. Research is summarized for factors that may cause one worker to be more or less prone to hearing loss than another. The reader is referred to Chasin (1996) for an in-depth overview of nonoccupational factors and issues.

TEMPORARY AND PERMANENT THRESHOLD SHIFTS

Most of the studies on the subject of threshold shifts relate to hearing loss in large-scale field studies and from experiments with animal models. The most common type of experiment is to elicit a temporary hearing loss referred to as a *temporary threshold shift* (TTS). As the name implies, TTS is the temporary elevation of the hearing threshold at one or more of the test frequencies and can be thought of as an early warning sign for a potentially *permanent threshold shift* (PTS). Most individuals have experienced TTS after a noisy day at work or even after a noisy rock concert. A feeling of numbness or dullness in the ears is perceived for a number of hours after the event and there may be an associated tinnitus or ringing in the ears for a period of time. If an individual's hearing is assessed immediately after such a noise event, a temporary sensorineural hearing loss may be found, which typically resolves in 16–18 hours.

TTS typically occurs at approximately one-half octave above the stimulus frequency and, as noted in Chapter 2, this would be in the 3000–6000 Hz region for most noise sources and for many forms of music. For very low-frequency stimuli (below 500 Hz), the region of TTS would be in the 300–750 Hz band regardless of exact stimulus frequency (Mills, Osguthorpe, Burdick, Patterson, & Mozo, 1983).

The relationship between TTS and PTS is not well defined, but it would be useful to examine some known correspondences. If a relationship were established, TTS could be used as a predictor of PTS. In 1966, the Committee on Hearing and Bioacoustics (CHABA) attempted to establish a model that would define the relationship between TTS and PTS . In the words of CHABA, "If any single band exceeds the damage-risk contours specified, the noise can be considered as potentially unsafe" (Kryter, Ward, Miller, & Eldredge, 1966).

Because of the gaps in information and lack of a firm theoretical basis, CHABA made several assumptions in order to obtain the resulting damage risk contours. One such simplifying assumption was that the recovery from TTS is related only to the magnitude of the TTS— the larger the TTS, the longer it takes to resolve. However, subsequent research demonstrated that "recovery from TTS depends on both the duration and the intensity of the noise exposure" (Melnick, 1991, p. 149).

Another implicit assumption was that intermittent noise with regular quiet periods would be less damaging than steady state noise. But how quiet do the spaces in between the noise bursts have to be for there to be a reduction in the level of damage? Ward, Cushing, & Burns (1976) developed upper limit estimates of *effective quiet* (a level that would produce no TTS) and these were significantly quieter than the estimates CHABA utilized for its damage risk contours. These are shown in Table 3–1.

Mills, Gilbert, and Adkins (1979) also calculated *critical levels*, which are those octave band intensities that would cause 5 dB of TTS after 16

TABLE 3–1. Estimates of "Effective Quiet" in dB SPL for Different Studies

Frequency	Ward et al. (1976)	Mills et al. (1979)	Ranges from 7 Studies Cited in Mills et al. (1979)
250	77	—	—
500	76	82	75–85
1000	69	82	81–82
2000	68	78	77–78
4000	65	74	74–76
Broadband	76 dBA	78 dBA	

hours. These authors summarized the results of seven earlier studies of critical levels on humans which can also be found in Table 3–1. The data from Ward, Cushing, and Burns (1976) and Mills, Gilbert, and Adkins (1979) are remarkably similar, once corrected for the difference in definition between effective quiet and critical level.

Intermittence and fluctuating noise add to the difficulty in establishing damage risk criteria. The variability in the intensity of some noise sources can be thought of as "on times" and "off times," with the on times being those that are more intense. The CHABA damage risk contours (Kryter et al., 1966) utilize a relationship referred to as the *on fraction rule* "[that] predicts that when the noise is on for half of the total period of exposure, the amount of TTS would be one-half of that which would have been produced if the noise had been continuous" (Melnick, 1991, p. 150). There have been some criticisms of this relationship but they pertain to longer on times than 2–3 minutes and for spectra with significant low-frequency energy below 1200 Hz (Selters & Ward, 1962; Melnick, 1991).

Whether the full benefit of intermittent noise (or music) can be achieved or not, undoubtedly some relief is provided, but its exact magnitude cannot be precisely ascertained. "If it is possible to venture any general conclusion . . . [it is that] intermittence does reduce hazard" (Ward, 1991, p. 168).

The relationship between PTS and TTS is not simple. Although some individuals may appear to be prone to hearing loss from noise or music exposure as evidenced in a large PTS or long recovery time from TTS, the correlation is very low when group data are taken (Taylor, Pearson, Mair, & Burns, 1965; Henderson, Hamernik, & Sitler, 1974; Henderson, Subramaniam, & Boettcher, 1993). One can say, however, that if noise does not cause TTS, then it will also not cause PTS (U.S. Department of Labor, 1981; Henderson et al., 1993).

Ward (1970) suggested that an examination of recovery time from TTS may provide a better index of predicting PTS as long as the noise is of high intensity and high frequency. Such a noise spectrum is commonly found in the case of rock drummers and others in their immediate vicinity, as well as in the workers exposed to many forms of impulse noise, such as in stamping plants. A longitudinal study of such musicians and workers might provide some reliable predictive data.

MODELS OF PTS

Between 1968 and 1973 there were a number of field studies on the relationship between noise exposure and PTS (Passchier-Vermeer, 1968, 1971; Robinson, 1968, 1971; Baughn, 1973; Lempert & Henderson, 1973).

Indeed, the Passchier-Vermeer, Robinson, and Baughn studies formed the basis of the 1973 U.S. Environmental Protection Agency's (Environmental Protection Agency, 1973) Criteria Document and noted very little PTS for noise levels below 85 dBA if an individual were exposed for 8 hours per day for 40 years. It should be pointed out that this is for the average PTS measured at 500 Hz, 1000 Hz, and 2000 Hz. Although these studies had good correlation at these midrange frequencies, the agreement was poorer for 4000 Hz, especially for the higher exposure levels.

The Lempert and Henderson (1973) study formed the basis of the National Institute for Occupational Safety and Health (NIOSH, 1973) model and is in good agreement with the previous studies at lower exposure levels, but tended to predict a greater PTS at higher exposure levels if measured at 500 Hz, 1000 Hz, and 2000 Hz.

A more recent model is based on the International Organization for Standardization (ISO) (1990) standard R-1999, which appears to be in good agreement with the previous models. Indeed "models such as ISO R-1999 are sufficiently accurate to support the needs of most regulators, administrators, and others who need rough predictions on the effects of noise on groups of workers" (Johnson, 1991, p. 174). In their study of noise exposure for railway workers, Henderson and Saunders (1998) concluded that "growth of hearing loss can be projected fairly well based on ISO 1999, without knowledge of the details of spectrum or level of noise exposure" (p. 120). The ISO does state emphatically that "group results cannot and should not be used at any time when an individual is considered" (Glorig & Linthicum, 1998, p. 54).

There have been some criticisms of ISO R-1999 and these mostly revolve around the interaction between noise exposure and the effects of presbycusis (Bies & Hansen, 1990; Macrae, 1991; Bies, 1994; Mills, Boettcher, & Dubno, 1997; Glorig & Linthicum, 1998; Ward, 1998). For younger workers these criticisms should not be a factor, however. At the other end of the scale, Rosenhall, Pedersen, and Svanborg (1990) showed that, by age 79, there was no longer a difference between those who had been exposed to noise and those who had not. That is, eventually presbycusis becomes a much more dominant factor.

Related to the Rosenhall et al. (1990) data, an interesting feature regarding the progression of PTS over time can be seen in Figure 3–1. Even though the ISO R-1999 standard has data only for noise exposures greater than 10 years, by using some of the studies that ISO R-1999 are based on (Burns & Robinson, 1970; Passchier-Vermeer, 1968) one can predict a greater rate of increase in PTS over the first few years of noise exposure than in subsequent years. Early education regarding the potential effects of noise (and recreational noise) is therefore imperative. An alternative way of looking at the same data is that, by the time a

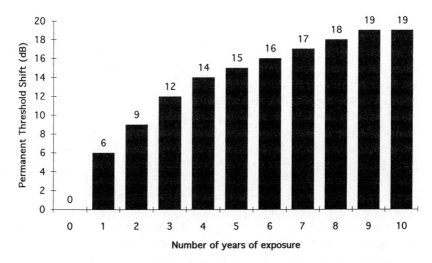

Figure 3-1. Predicted permanent hearing loss over time by the ISO R-1999 model. A greater rate of PTS is predicted over the first few years of noise exposure than in subsequent years.

worker seeks audiological advice, the progression of hearing loss may have slowed and this would be useful in counseling the worker that he or she "will not go deaf."

Whenever several large scale studies are combined into one model, caution needs to be exercised. As pointed out by Henderson and Saunders (1998), in the case of ISO R-1999, the Burns and Robinson (1970) study used subjects who were vigorously screened and were only exposed to continuous noise, whereas the Passchier-Vermeer (1968) study used subjects who were exposed to both impact and continuous noise. Another concern involves the boundary or start conditions of the model: Do 18-year-old, nonexposed men have a hearing loss? Ward (1998) stated that, "Even Robinson, who is responsible for incorporation of the erroneous equating of age correction and HTL into ISO 1999, is now willing to admit that any real-world sample of 18-year-old males will show median HTLs of 3–6 dB" (p. 19).

Table 3–2 summarizes the 4000 Hz PTS of these studies at three exposure levels (85 dBA, 90 dBA, and 95 dBA). There are no large databases for exposures levels below 85 dBA, and while some data indicate a small PTS after a number of years for exposure levels as low as 75 dBA (Robinson, 1968, 1971), and a small TTS (Mills et al., 1979), nonoccupational sources of noise and music exposure can become very significant. It would be impossible to factor these nonoccupational sources into a model with any degree of certainty or accuracy. Recreational noise is cer-

TABLE 3-2. Summary of Five Studies on Predicted Permanent Threshold Shift (in dB) at 4000 Hz for Three Exposure Levels

Intensity	Passchier-Vermeer (1971)	Robinson (1968)	Baughn (1973)	NIOSH (1973)	ISO R-1999 (1990)
85 dBA	8	6	9	5	6
90 dBA	15	12	14	11	11
95 dBA	23	18	17	20	21

tainly one factor (Clark, 1991b; Johnson, 1991; Chasin, 1996), but the long-term effects have not yet been established.

IMPULSE NOISE AND MODELS

Most of the models of noise-induced hearing loss are adequate for levels up to 115 dBA; however, they tend to break down for more intense impulse stimuli such as some impulse noise sources. Price and Kalb (1991) and Price (1994) investigated the effects of intense impulse sounds and found that the motion of the basilar membrane during the impulse sound was also important for the prediction of hearing loss (other than intensity and duration). Price (1994) noted that, "at lower SPLs losses are in all likelihood largely a function of the metabolic demand on the inner ear (it gets 'tired out') and that above some spectrally dependent critical level, the loss mechanism changes to one of mechanical disruption . . . (the ear gets 'torn up')." He argues that if the basilar membrane is allowed to oscillate past the zero (atmospheric pressure) point, then more damage will be sustained by the hair cells in the organ of Corti. If impulses possess either completely positive or completely negative pressure waves, the displacement of the middle ear ossicles cannot impart sufficient energy to create a "tearing" action to the inner ear structures.

Although a cap pistol (at 30 cm) and two small wooden blocks (impacting at 2 cm) have almost identical peak sound pressure levels (150–153 dB SPL), because of the shape of the pressure wave, the small wooden blocks would cause a 25 dB permanent hearing loss but the cap pistol would only cause a 10 dB permanent hearing loss.

PTS AND EXCHANGE RATES

The damage risk contours discussed in the CHABA document refer to contours of equal risk of permanent hearing loss given a specified intensity and specified duration of exposure. That is, a relationship exists between the exposure sound level and length of exposure time. This relationship is called the *exchange rate*. A 3-dB exchange rate (or 3-dB rule) means that there is an identical risk if the sound level is increased by 3 dB, but for only half the amount of time of exposure. A 3-dB exchange rate would imply that the risk for damage doubles every 3 dB (or, equivalently, decreases by half for every decrease of 3 dB). A 5-dB exchange rate implies that risk doubles for every 5 dB increase in exposure level.

Correspondences can be derived with exchange rates. For example, a 3-dB exchange rate would state that the damage of a 95 dBA noise level for 8 hours is identical to the damage from 98 dBA for 4 hours, or the damage from 107 dBA for only 30 minutes. A 5-dB exchange rate would be more conservative: 95 dBA for 8 hours causes the same damage as 100 dBA for 4 hours or 115 dBA for only 30 minutes. Thus, a 5-dB exchange rate would predict a lower risk than a 3-dB exchange rate.

The relationship of the PTS due to steady state noise to the PTS due to fluctuating noise is complicated, but some researchers (Martin, 1976; Robinson, 1976) have argued that fluctuating noise can be equally as hazardous as a steady state noise of "equal energy." Proponents of the *equal energy hypothesis* would advocate a 3-dB exchange rate.

However, many TTS experiments and researchers, such as Ward (1976, 1998) have argued that noises that produce equal amounts of TTS are equally damaging. Proponents of this point of view would advocate a 5-dB exchange rate.

Embleton (1995), in reporting on the results of an International Institute of Noise Control Engineering Working Party paper, concluded that, "the scientific evidence is that 3 dB is probably the most reasonable exchange rate for daily noise exposure. Statistically it is also a good approximation for the results of many epidemological studies relating to intermittent exposures, even though these show considerable spread about any mean curve" (p. 18).

In contrast, Dear (1998) argues for a 5-dB exchange rate, stating that much of the background for the 3-dB exchange rate derives from the Burns and Robinson (1970) study, which he finds to be flawed. He lists over 20 criticisms of the Burns and Robinson data, citing issues of poor experimental design, misinterpretation of data, and conclusions that are more advocacy than scholarship.

It should be emphasized that these exchange rates are meant only to summarize data and they can be an oversimplification (Ward, 1976). Indeed, Johnson (1973) noted that, as a convenient data summarizing tool, the 5-dB exchange rate seems to be appropriate for hearing losses in the mid frequencies (500 Hz to 2000 Hz) and the 3-dB exchange rate is more appropriate for 4000 Hz. Finally, Ward (1974, 1982) pointed out that the effects of noise exposure are caused by dosage and not merely by sound level.

AUDITORY TOUGHENING OR
THE TRAINING EFFECT

First noted by Miller, Watson, and Covell (1963), *auditory toughening* or the *training effect*, is the auditory system's ability to modify its susceptibility to damage from noise, depending on previous exposures. Specifically, when the auditory system is "toughened" by nondamaging exposure to noise for a number of days, ensuing hearing loss as a result of a damaging level of spectrally similar noise is *less* than that which would occur if there was no previous toughening.

This phenomenon has been observed for PTS in a wide range of mammals as well as for TTS among teenagers (Miyakita, Hellstrom, Frimansson, & Axelsson, 1992). Figure 3–2 indicates that, after a toughening or training of the ear for 10 days to a 500 Hz band of noise (even after a 5-day period of recovery), a smaller PTS was found than in chinchillas that were not toughened.

However, this experiment was for chinchillas that were toughened and later exposed to high levels of the same noise (e.g., 500 Hz). Subramanian, Henderson, and Spongr (1991) examined the effects on a low-frequency toughening (500 Hz) but a high-frequency exposure (4000 Hz). In this case, the reverse result was obtained—the toughening actually increased the PTS over that of the nontoughened or control group.

In summary, it seems that if the nondamaging toughening stimulus is the same as the more traumatic one presented later, then there will be some protection from this effect. However, if the toughening stimulus is low-frequency and the traumatic one is high frequency, then the high-frequency effect may exacerbate the hearing loss.

The process of auditory toughening or the training effect is not well understood. Hamernik and Ahroon (1998) suggested that, "the operative mechanism for any protective effect is that associated with the spreading of energy over time rather than a toughening of the cochlea" (p. 3487). Thus a toughened cochlea is not necessarily one that is more protected against noise exposure. Possible explanations may be related

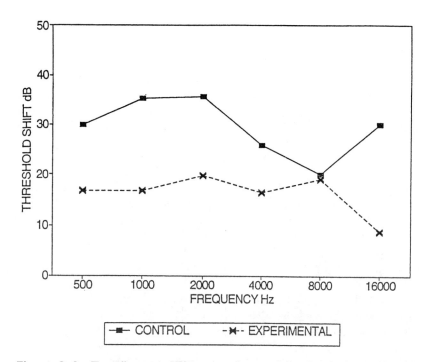

Figure 3-2. The difference in PTS between the experimental group that received 10 days of "conditioning" exposures, and a control group after a 48 hour exposure to 500 Hz at 106 dB SPL. (Reprinted with permission from "Individual Susceptibility to Noise–Induced Hearing Loss," by D. Henderson, M. Subramian, and F. A. Boettcher, 1993. *Ear and Hearing, 14,* 152–168.

to the effects of the efferent neurological pathways and the effects of the presence of proteins in the outer hair cells (Zheng, Henderson, McFadden, & Hu, 1997). More research on this topic is required.

HEARING LOSS AND INDIVIDUAL FACTORS

Studies in the research literature are inconclusive with respect to evidence for an altered susceptibility of hearing loss based on individual factors such as melanin levels, eye color, and sex.

Robinson (1988) found weak statistical evidence that eye color is related to hearing loss, but only for certain frequencies, and the available sample sizes are small. Similar results previously had been found by Carter (1980) and by Carlin and McCrosky (1980). Generally, blue-eyed people were found to be more susceptible to hearing loss from noise exposure than those with more melanin content in their eyes. Cooper (1994), in commenting on Robinson's work, found that most of Robinson's groups had statistical sampling problems that limited the validity of the conclusions. Nevertheless, Henselman et al. (1995), in studying U.S. Army soldiers, found a significant difference in hearing levels "among the race groups with black soldiers having the most sensitive hearing and white soldiers having the poorest" (p. 382).

Cooper (1994) did, however, find that older women generally have poorer low-frequency hearing sensitivity and this may be related to estrogen and its relationship to metabolic presbycusis. At higher frequencies, Cooper noted that men had worse hearing thresholds than women, when matched for age. Berger, Royster, and Thomas (1978) also found that men had worse hearing thresholds than age-matched women when exposed to equivalent levels of noise over a number of years. Johnson (1991) attributed much of this difference to the level of nonoccupational noise exposure that men are subject to relative to that of women.

Henderson et al. (1993) noted that, although genetic factors such as eye color and sex are significant in well-controlled studies, they account for only a small fraction of the variability in studies on hearing loss. Borg and his colleagues (Borg, Canlon, & Engström, 1995) listed eight sources of individual variability and these are given in Table 3–3.

TABLE 3–3. Sources of Individual Variability of Permanent Noise Induced Hearing Loss.

---

1. Inappropriate description of exposure conditions.

2. Variability of hearing protection usage.

3. Individual sound transmission of the ear (including ear canal, middle ear, and stapedial reflex).

4. Individual susceptibility of the inner ear structures (including hair cells, supporting structures, and membranes).

5. Physiological factors such as function of inner ear, blood flow, inner ear chemistry, and efferent feedback.

6. Other non-noise-induced causes such as hereditary factors, toxins, aging, and infections.

7. Interaction with other ergonomic factors such as vibration, temperature, work load, toxins, and radiation.

8. Errors in determining hearing threshold (including tester error, response error, and temporary conditions such as TTS).

Source: Adapted with permission from "Noise Induced Hearing Loss" by E. Borg, B. Canlon, & B. Engstrom, 1995, *Scandinavian Audiology,* Suppl. 40, p. 33. Copyright 1995 by Scandinavian University Press.

OXYGEN SUPPLY AND HEARING LOSS

A small but growing body of research is attempting to answer the exact nature of the interaction between hearing loss and an increased carbon monoxide level (or decreased oxygen supply) such as that found with smoking tobacco (see, for example, Chung, Wilson, Gannon, & Mason, 1982; Prince & Matonoski, 1991; Barone, Peters, Garabrant, Bernstein, & Krebsbach, 1987). However, no definitive study provides conclusive evidence. This is probably related to the fact that those who smoke also have other physiological problems that may alter their susceptibility to hearing loss from noise exposure. Further, interactions exist that (depending on the factors and their levels) may increase or decrease an individual's propensity for hearing loss.

There is evidence that cardiovascular function (Sanden & Axelsson, 1981) and overall physical fitness (Ismail et al., 1973) can affect the propensity for hearing loss. Sanden and Axelsson found that shipyard workers with greater increases in heart rate and blood pressure when working hard had the greatest hearing losses. Ismail et al. studied the degree of TTS initially and after the same subjects completed an 8-month physical training program and found that after the training program there was significantly less TTS.

Vittitow, Windmill, Yates, and Cunningham (1994) discussed two physiological processes in order to explain the interaction between noise exposure and poor oxygen supply to the cochlea. The first is metabolic exhaustion and this "occurs when a hair cell [in the cochlea] fails to convert nutrients and expel waste in accordance with the stress demands placed upon it" (p. 347). When nutrients such as oxygen are not adequately supplied, hair cell damage occurs. The other process is vascular (Lawrence, Gonzales, & Hawkins, 1967, 1971); noise may damage the vascular structures of the cochlea, thereby cutting off the oxygen supply route to the hair cells. The vascular process is controversial and more research needs to be performed.

More recently, using a sophisticated computer-controlled technique, Goldwyn, Khan, Shivapuja, Seidman, and Quirk (1998) examined the vascular cochlear microcirculation changes as a result of noise exposure. They found that, "Exposures to noise resulted in alterations in cochlear microcirculation that produced localized ischemia in the stria vascularis [lining] of the cochlear wall" (p. 581). Goldwyn and his colleagues feel that some of the inconclusive results of previous studies may have been related to inappropriate noise levels, inappropriate animal models, and nonsensitive microcirculatory assessment techniques.

Hétu, Phaneuf, and Marien (1987), in reviewing some studies on the acute and chronic effects of carbon monoxide, found reduced performance on auditory perception tasks and concluded that the major site of lesion was the auditory cortex. Patchett (1992) found that inhalation of oxygen during noise exposure reduces TTS.

Hearing loss from noise exposure is undoubtedly related to a combination of these processes (and sites of lesion) and indicates that excessive levels of carbon monoxide and/or lower levels of oxygen in the bloodstream would increase one's susceptibility to noise exposure. However, Dengerink, Trueblood, and Dengerink (1984) found that the effects of smoking and cold temperatures *decreased* one's susceptibility to hearing loss. They argued that both of these factors cause a *peripheral* vasoconstriction, thereby increasing the blood flow to more central locations such as the cochlea. Dengerink, Lindgren, Axelsson, and Dengerink (1987) also found that exercise *and* smoking in noise decreased susceptibility to hearing loss as compared with a nonsmoking, nonexercising group. It was argued that more blood supply was available to the central locations such as the cochlea of the smokers because of the peripheral vasoconstriction of this group. In this same vein, they also found that lower body temperature decreased susceptibility to noise exposure.

These findings are not necessarily contradictory. Simply stated, if there is less oxygen and/or more carbon monoxide (from smoking) available to the cochlea, there will be an increased susceptibility to noise exposure. The above studies support the contention that factors affecting the cardiovascular system may have a major effect on the auditory system.

There is a growing list of chemical interactions that, depending on the environment, may alter susceptibility to noise exposure in an occupational setting. The reader is referred to excellent reviews by Hétu, et al. (1987) and by Boettcher, Henderson, Gratton, Danielson, and Byrne (1987) for in-depth information.

NONAUDITORY EFFECTS OF NOISE EXPOSURE

Nonauditory effects of noise exposure are effects that do not cause hearing loss, but which nevertheless have other real effects. Some of these effects are seen by a change in body functions, such as heart rate, and in learning/cognition in children. Nonauditory effects of noise exposure were noted as early as 1930 (Smith & Laird, 1930). In that study, nonauditory effects pertain to stomach contractions in healthy human beings when exposed to noise.

Similar to the research concerning the auditory effects of noise, there are both laboratory studies and field studies of nonauditory effects. In laboratory studies, well controlled conditions are set up, using paradigms that seek to control certain variables. Laboratory studies are therefore more suited to examining changes in certain measures, but are typically unsuited for examining long-term effects that may result in disease or cognitive/educational problems (Bronzaft, 1991). Although laboratory studies can be more precise than field studies, they may or may not have any bearing on reality. In contrast, field studies are inherently less well designed to control for unwanted variables, but their conclusions may be more applicable to reality. Field studies are well suited to look at the long-term effects of disease and/or educational affects. A major difficulty with all research into nonauditory factors is that subjective responses not based on intensity or duration may be quite significant. Three classic studies from the early 1980s that provide an excellent overview for the interested reader are: Thompson (1981), Cohen and Weinstein (1981), and DeJoy (1984).

Cardiovascular Effects of Noise

Most of the studies on cardiovascular effects have been performed in the laboratory, on animals. Many of the early studies were performed by assessing blood pressure in rats. Rats have been used in the past because of their low cost of maintenance and acquisition. However DeJoy (1984) commented that the rat may not be an appropriate model, and that a primate species may be more appropriate. It was found that, indeed, when primates are used as an animal model, as noise level increased so did blood pressure, but there is still a large degree of variability in the studies.

In the few field studies on humans, blood pressure was also the measurement tool, but again the level of variability was great. Sloan (1991), while reviewing available data, noted that, when taken as a whole, "although there are inconsistencies in the findings . . . they generally support the assertion that exposure to noise is associated with higher levels of blood pressure" (p. 23). Data are still limited however, and the results may depend on many uncontrolled factors, such as subjective response, the exact nature of physiological assessment, and the animal model. In addition, it is still not known if increased blood pressure in a noisy environment will lead to cardiovascular disease.

The physiological rationales of the effects on body chemistry as a result of increased exposure to noise are beyond the scope of this book, but the interested reader is referred to Raymond (1991). In summarizing several studies he noted many methodological problems, but also noted an overall increase in total serum cholesterol level in some workers when exposed to noise levels in excess of 80 dBA (in addition to an increase in diastolic blood pressure, even though there was no increase in the systolic blood pressure and heart rate).

Sleep Effects of Noise

Pollak (1991) noted that "noises are more annoying when they occur at times when people expect to rest or sleep, (2) noise can interrupt sleep, and (3) noise can also have subtle effects on sleep . . . that are detectable only with specialized instruments" (p. 41). Most laboratory studies use truck and aircraft noise as stimuli and measure the effect on a range of sleep study parameters. Noise can delay sleep, and shift the sleep stages upward (i.e., more shallow sleeping). Upward sleep stage shifts have been observed even in relative quiet with changes noted for stimuli as quiet as 25–30 dB SPL. Cardiovascular changes are usually not noted until the stimulus level is just below the arousal level for that individual. Thiessen (1978, 1983) found that, as peak noise intensity increased, there was a linear increase in the probability of a change in sleep stage.

Some groups appear to have their sleep patterns adversely effected by noise levels that would have minimal effect on other groups. Among the former are chronic and acute care patients in hospitals, the elderly, and shift workers. Frese and Harwich (1984) noted in shift workers that factors such as nonoccupational noise, coffee, and smoking were all predictive indicators of daytime sleep disturbance.

Effects of Noise on Fetal Development

There are some data suggesting an increased risk of noise-induced damage in fetuses, but this is still a very controversial issue. The interested reader is referred to Ryals (1990) for more information.

Nakamura (1977) noted low birth weights when the pregnant mother was exposed to high levels of occupational noise. Schell (1981) found that noise may in fact decrease birth weight. However, Edmonds, Layde, and Erickson (1979), in a well controlled field study, found that when exposed to aircraft noise, there was no significant data suggesting that noise could affect fetal development in pregnant women.

Effects of Noise on Learning

When speech is masked by background noise (as it can be in a noisy party), this is similar to having a hearing loss (with equivalent masked hearing thresholds). Children with even slight hearing losses have been shown to have decreased educational and cognitive performance. Davis (1985) found that children with a minimal (25 dB) hearing loss scored almost two full grade levels lower in reading comprehension by grade 4 (despite having minimal differences in grade 1). This is equivalent to normal hearing children being subject to environmental noise levels of only 50–60 dBA in their hearing environment. Matkin (1988) found that the language delay as measured on certain language tests was 1–2 years depending on hearing loss (or equivalently significant environmental noise level).

Specifically with respect to normal hearing children in a noisy school environment, Cohen, Glass, and Singer (1973) found that children whose classrooms were on the street level (nearer to truck and car noise) performed poorer on reading ability tasks than children whose classrooms were in quieter locations. Bronzaft and McCarthy (1975) studied the reading ability of children in one school near elevated train tracks. Half of the classrooms faced the train track and the other half were on the quieter back part of the school. Students in the quieter classrooms did better on reading achievement tests, and by grade 6, those in the quieter classrooms were a full grade point ahead of those in the noisier classrooms. Green, Pasternak, and Shore (1982), in studying children near a New York airport, found that, as noise level increased, the percentage of those children falling below grade reading level also increased. Finally, Wachs (1982) noted that children were slower to develop language skills in noisier homes.

A FINAL WORD

Many factors potentially can affect hearing ability. And not all people are as equally susceptible to hearing loss from these factors. Therefore, caution should always be exercised when drawing conclusions about the effects for any one individual. With any degree of certainty one can only make statements about groups of worker, and when other factors are controlled for. The topic of the effects of nonauditory noise exposure—exposure that manifests itself in other non-hearing-related ways—is still very much in its infancy. Research that is both valid and reliable is very difficult to perform. Because of the inherent differences in real-world situations and well controlled laboratory situations, data need to be interpreted with caution. Nevertheless, nonauditory factors have been noted and can play an important part in the development and well being of people.

4

Noise Measurement

hapter 1 described the main characteristics of sound, such as sound pressure, power, intensity, frequency content, and so on, but did not specifically examine how those characteristics are measured. The objective of this chapter is to explain the basic instruments and techniques used for measuring noise.

The accuracy of a measurement result is related not only to the accuracy of the instrumentation but also to the technique used. For example, the obvious way to measure the speed of a car is to measure the time it takes to go from a point A to a point B. Then, by dividing the distance by the time, one can easily obtain the speed. However, the accuracy of this determination will be strongly influenced by the way (and the accuracy) the distance has been measured. More important yet, the result will depend on the way the time is measured, the instrument used, and whether the instances when the car was passing through both points were determined by optical means or just by a naked eye. Such factors will influence the result of the measurement in such a way that another person using a different method (and/or instrumentation) could obtain different results.

There are several ways of defining how a measurement should be performed. Usually the manuals provided with the instruments give some guidance on this issue. When the result of the measurement is needed to certify compliance with an official Bylaw or Act, then there will be detailed descriptions not only of the procedure to be followed, but also of the precautions to be taken and how the report should be prepared.

Finally, there are the official measurement standards issued by a national or international institution. These are documents of higher quality, where the instrumentation to be used and the way measurements are to be performed are defined so that persons performing the same measurement at different locations and/or using different instruments will obtain the same result if they follow the same procedure.

In Canada, the Canadian Standards Association (CSA), a nongovernmental body, publishes measurement standards. In the U.S.A. this is done by the American National Standards Institute (ANSI). On the international scene, the International Organization for Standardization (ISO), located in Geneva, publishes the international standards, written by experts from the different participating countries.

Such principles apply equally for measuring noise: depending on the technique being followed, the results of a given measurement can be substantially different. That is why this chapter deals with both instruments and procedures.[1]

THE BASIC INSTRUMENT

What has been called the *basic instrument* helps to understand the instrumentation that will be described further in this chapter. It contains the essential elements that every acoustical instrument has: see Figure 4–1.

All acoustical instruments are electronic devices. Because sound is essentially a mechanical phenomenon, there is a need for a transducer, a device capable of transforming the acoustical signal, which is mechanical in nature, into an electronic signal that can be later analyzed, transformed, and so on. The device that transforms the mechanical movement of the air molecules into an electrical signal is the *microphone.*

There are many types of microphones. They are designed for different purposes. Some are simple devices used at home for entertaining. There are also the professional types used mainly for the broadcasting/ TV industry. Finally, there are the precision microphones used for acoustical measurements. The differences among microphones are in the accuracy in the transduction process, the dynamic range (sound level range they can operate within without distortion), temperature and humidity ranges and so on. Since most acoustical instruments are of the precision type they make use of high quality microphones that must be able to maintain their accuracy even in extreme environmental conditions. The microphone is one of the most expensive and delicate parts of many acoustical instruments. That is why it should be handled with extreme care.

Once the acoustical signal has been transformed into an electrical one, it is introduced into the *signal processor,* which is specific for the use of the particular instrument. Basically, processors are electronic devices. Some are very sophisticated and semiautomatic. Others have controls that are handled by the instrument operator.

---

[1]The terms "technique" and "procedure" are used as synonyms in this chapter.

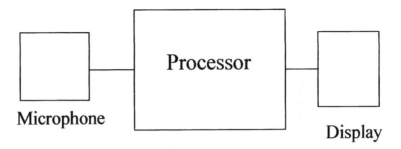

Figure 4–1. The basic instrument.

Finally, the result of the measurement is shown on a *display*, which can be either analog or digital. In some cases, there are even instruments whose display is graphic, but that applies to specific cases of relatively expensive devices.

Most instruments have output connections that allow the signal to be sent to peripheral devices such as printers, tape recorders, and computers.

THE SOUND LEVEL METER (SLM)

The SLM is the basic and also the most often used instrument for acoustical measurements. Its use covers a wide range of applications, including the measurement of occupational, recreational, and environmental noise.

There is a wide variety of SLMs, depending on their precision, the data that can be obtained and the way they are displayed. However, all have to conform with national or international standards and this fact has to be included in their instruction manuals, where their characteristics are shown.

It is highly recommended that the manual provided by the manufacturer be carefully examined once an instrument has been purchased. This is the best way for the operator to become familiar with the controls and how to properly handle and care for the device. Another good practice for users is to consult the manual every time they perform a measurement, until they feel confident in the instrument's operation.

A block diagram of a SLM is shown in Figure 4–2 and a photograph of an actual instrument is shown in Figure 4–3.

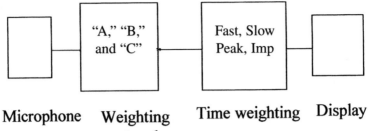

Microphone   Weighting   Time weighting   Display
                network

Figure 4-2. Block diagram of a SLM.

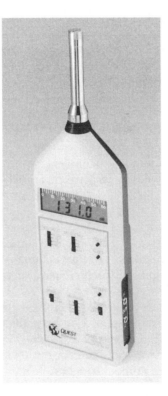

Figure 4-3. Sound level meter.

The Microphone

As with the basic instrument described earlier, sound is detected by a microphone, which is usually part of the body of the instrument. However, many types of SLMs have the option of connecting the microphone to a cable, so that it can be located away from the instrument. This is done in situations where the operator cannot be located close to the sound source because of his personal safety or to prevent his physical presence from influencing the measurement.

The Weighting Networks

The signal is processed in two different ways. The first is using the three weighting networks (filters) "A", "B," and "C," which were discussed in Chapter 1. As shown in Figure 1–8, the filter "A" greatly attenuates the lower frequencies, especially frequencies lower than 500 Hz, while the use of filter "C" leaves almost all of the acoustical energy as is, without any attenuation. These characteristics provide some idea of the frequency distribution of a signal. If most of the energy is contained in the lower end of the spectrum, then the reading on the display using the "A" filter will be much lower than when using the "C" filter. On the other hand, if most of the energy is in the upper end, then there will be little or no difference when measuring in dBA [2] or in dBC.

In summary, if the reading in dBA is similar to the one in dBC, then most of the energy is contained in the upper region of the spectrum. The opposite is also valid: A reading in dBA that is much lower than in dBC indicates that most of the energy is concentrated in the lower end of the spectrum.

Changing from one filter to other is done manually using a knob, a button, or a sliding switch, depending on the make of the SLM. One has to be careful in knowing which setting is being used for the measurement, because the readings will be quite different depending on the filter being used.

When no filter is desired, the filter selector in many SLMs has a position that eliminates all three filters and the signal is processed without any change in its frequency content. Readings made without using a weighting network are expressed as dBLin.

---

[2]As mentioned in Chapter 1, a measurement performed using filter "A" is expressed in dBA. The same applies when the other two filters (B and C) are used: results will be expressed as dBB and dBC respectively.

The Time Response

Before the signal reaches the display, another process takes place: determining how the signal should be shown on the display. Most signals are highly variable with time. Even if they are not impulsive or interrupted, their amplitude changes continuously. One example of a variable noise is traffic noise, where the sound level increases or decreases with each car that passes close to the observer. Another is noise in an office, resulting from ringing of phones, conversations, traffic, and office machines.

If a rapidly changing signal is presented on the display, we will see numbers that will continuously change and it will thus be almost impossible to determine the actual noise level at that particular place.

A solution to this problem is a time-integrating filter, known as the *Slow* setting, which provides a kind of average level of the variable noise. The time constant of the filter, as per the applicable standards, is 1 second. Its effect is to "slow down" the variations of what is read on the display.

The Slow setting is used most frequently, since all national and international standards require that noise be measured in this way whenever the object is to assess occupational, environmental, and/or recreational activities.

In some situations (such as when measuring the maximum noise level emitted by a passing vehicle) one is interested in the maximum values of the sound level. Another filter—the *Fast* one—is used in this case. Its frequency response is only 125 ms in duration.

Impulse noises have a very short duration (less than 0.5 s) with a pause between two consecutive impulses of at least 0.5 s. The characteristic measured in this kind of noise is the *peak*, defined as the maximum value attained by the sound level. A special kind of SLM, known as *Impulse SLM* (ISLM), can measure the peak of such a noise. Such instruments have a special setting called *Peak*. The time constant of this setting is of 50 microseconds. The result of measuring the peak of an impulse noise is expressed in dB_{Peak}.

Finally, there is the *Impulse* setting, with a time constant of 35 ms. It has very limited applications, and is used mainly for assessing the annoyance of impulsive noise.

The Battery Check

SLMs are battery operated. Since the life of batteries is limited, the operator needs to know their state and replace them when needed. In some older models, a button has to be pressed to have the state of the battery displayed.

Most modern SLMs get the indication of a low battery directly, without having to perform any operation. Because the use of a SLM with low batteries will show results that are not reliable, batteries should be checked before and after each series of measurements.

Internal Calibration

All SLMs provide for a check of the entire electronic circuit of the instrument. To do so, an electrical signal is injected at the microphone output. The manufacturer indicates the reading that should appear on the display. A calibration control allows for adjusting that particular reading to the value that it is supposed to indicate.

This internal calibration assures the operator that the instrument is in proper condition, ready to be used. There is, however, a drawback in the fact that this internal signal is injected after the microphone, allowing for the control of the entire electronic part of the instrument. The internal calibration will not show whether the microphone is out of order. That is done by using an acoustical calibrator that generates a sound to be applied directly to the microphone of the SLM, as it will be explained later in this chapter.

The Display

The display in most older SLMs is analog, with a logarithmic scale of $+10/-6$ dB range. The zero is located to the left on the scale. To make a reading, the attenuator of the instrument (that has steps of 10 dB), is adjusted so that the needle of the display is working primarily on the right side of the scale (i.e., above the 0 dB mark). The reading of the sound level is performed by adding the reading on the display to that on the attenuator.

For example, if the needle indicates 7 dB on the scale and the attenuator is set to 70 dB, then the measurement result will be $70 + 7 = 77$ dB. With the same setting of the attenuator, if the needle shows -2 dB, the measurement result will be $70 - 2 = 68$ dB.

Most newer SLMs make use of a digital display The reading is direct and there is no need to add the attenuator's indication to the reading. However, many SLMs still have attenuators that must be set to the proper range. The main advantage in this new technology is:

1. The attenuators now indicate ranges that are usually 60 dB or larger (i.e., they go between 30 and 90 dB, 40 and 100 dB, 50 and 110 dB, etc.), and
2. A warning is activated when the upper limit of the range has been exceeded.

For example, if the level to be measured is 105 and the range is 40–100, the display may still show 105 dB but an overload warning will appear on the display, indicating that the actual reading may not be correct and that there is a need for sliding the range further up, until the warning disappears.

THE INTEGRATING SLM (ISLM)

There are many different types of SLM, each with different precision or some special characteristics. One in particular is gaining popularity because of its capacity to measure the average sound level for as long as the operators wishes to. The Integrating SLM, as it is known, can perform all of the functions of an ordinary SLM. However, once it is set into the *Leq* mode, it provides a continuous reading of the average noise level from the time it is set to run. At the end of the measurement it also provides a reading of the duration time it had run.

The ISLM is particularly useful when assessing noise with a variable sound level and/or frequency content, the category most industrial, environmental, and office noises belong to.

All ISLMs have digital displays and, in most occasions, they are of the precision type. Because of those characteristics, their prices are higher than an ordinary SLM and the purchaser is advised to balance real needs with the uses for such an instrument.

THE CALIBRATOR

The calibrator is the instrument used for the complete calibration of the SLM, including the microphone. It consists of a small signal generator with a cavity that is applied directly over the microphone of the instrument to be calibrated.

Two types of calibrators are in actual use. One is the so-called *pistonphone*. It is a precision calibrator, where the signal is generated by the motion of a small piston driven by a battery energized motor. The sound pressure is obtained through the alternating motion of the piston. By carefully controlling the excursion, the amplitude (and hence the sound pressure level) is determined with very high accuracy ($+/- 0.15$ dB). The speed of the motor is proportional to the frequency of the signal and is also generated with high accuracy ($+/- 1\%$).

Because of the way the sound pressure is generated, pistonphones deliver 124 dB at 250 Hz. They are precision instruments and, as such, tend to be costly.

Much more popular are the acoustical calibrators (see Figure 4–4) that are pocket-sized, battery generated sound sources. Here the sound pressure is generated by a small loudspeaker, located in a cavity where the microphone of the instrument to be calibrated has to be introduced, in the same way as done with the previously described pistonphone. The use of a loudspeaker instead of a motor reduces both the accuracy (+ / − 0.3 dB in sound pressure and + / − 1.5% in frequency) and the cost of the calibrator. Even with lower accuracy, the calibrator is an excellent choice for most field applications.

Calibrators may generate more than one signal at more than one frequency. This is the direct consequence of the way the signals are generated. For instance, the calibrator in Figure 4–4 can provide signals with sound pressures of 94 dB and 114 dB at 250 and 1000 Hz. A wide variety of calibrators is available with models that generate signals at the octave frequencies between 125 and 8000 Hz and sound pressures between 40 and 110 dB in steps of 10 dB.

NOISE LEVEL MEASUREMENTS

It was pointed out previously that careful reading of the instrument's manual and a good knowledge of the instrument's operation are neces-

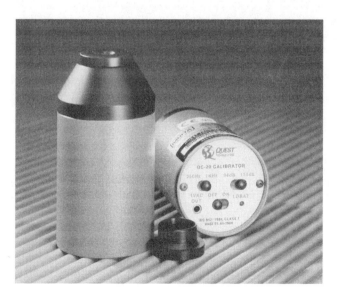

Figure 4–4. Calibrator.

sary conditions for performing a proper noise measurement. It is also advisable to find out if there is a regulation, bylaw, or standard that applies to the type of measurement to be performed. In many situations, precise protocols must be followed to obtain results considered reliable and acceptable by the appropriate authorities.

Most noise level measurements fall into two situations. In one, there are several sources and it is desired to determine which source contributes by how much to the resulting noise level. The second situation is related mostly to the assessment of the noise either at a workplace or residence to determine if the noise is hazardous, annoying, or work-interfering or if the measured level is in compliance with local laws or regulations.

In either situation, the measurement starts with checking the batteries and calibration of the SLM. The measurement should end with the same procedure to ensure that the instrument was in proper operating conditions during the entire measurement process.

Influence of the Background Noise

If the objective of the measurement is a noise source, another precaution must be taken to ensure that the background noise will not affect the results of the measurement. As discussed in Chapter 1, if the difference between the level measured with and without the source the background level is larger than 10 dB, then there is no need for corrections. On the other hand, if the difference is close to only 3 dB, then the result cannot possibly be known and the only way to determine it is to reduce the background noise and then perform the measurement again. For situations where the difference is between 3 and 10 dB, the measured level should be corrected using the values in Table 4–1.

The following four steps have to be done for the correction:

TABLE 4–1. Background noise correction.

Difference Between Levels	dB to be Subtracted from the Measured Level
≥10	0
6–9	1
4–5	2
3	3

1. Measure the source with the background noise present
2. Switch off the source and measure the background noise
3. Subtract the value of Step 2 from Step 1 and look for the appropriate correction from Table 4–1.
4. Subtract the correction from the value in Step 1. The result is the sound level of the source.

As an example, if the noise of the source (Step 1) is 93 dBA, and the background noise (Step 2) is 88 dBA, the difference will be 93 − 88 = 5 dBA, and the correction from Table 4–1 will be 2 dBA (Step 3). The actual noise level from the source will be 93 − 2 = 91 dBA (Step 4).

Care should be taken when reporting the measured levels. Most instruments allow for the measurement of levels with an accuracy of one decimal point. However, there is an uncertainty associated with field measurements of the order of ±2 dB. This is due to the fact that noises are seldom totally steady and there also are variations in the reading depending on the exact location of the microphone of the measuring instrument. Therefore, it is strongly recommended that the reading be rounded to the nearest integer (i.e., 3.4 = 3 and 3.6 = 4).

Microphone/Instrument Location

The microphone (or the whole instrument) should be kept away from the person holding it to minimize body reflections. The same precaution applies regarding reflecting walls and corners: Close proximity should be avoided. If possible, a tripod should be used to ensure that the instrument is steady and free from reflections. A standard height for the microphone during the measurements is 1.2 m (4 ft).

It is also recommended that, before taking the measurements, the microphone is moved up and down a couple of centimeters around the final microphone location to ensure that this location does not coincide with standing waves, which could lead to artificially high or low measuring results.

Influence of the Wind

When making measurements outdoors, the wind blowing against the microphone can also be a source of background noise, especially at high frequencies. To prevent measurement errors due to this effect, the use of a windscreen is recommended. This is a polyurethane foam sphere that fits around the microphone to reduce the wind effect; it also helps protect the microphone under dusty, oily, and wet conditions.

THE SOUND ANALYZER

Noise level measurements taken in dBA are most appropriate when assessing hazards, annoyance, work interference, and so on caused by noise. However, when the objective of the measurement is noise control, then the information given in dBA is not sufficient. The frequency content and distribution (e.g., the frequency spectrum) are also needed. The instrument that does this is the sound analyzer. Basically, this is a sound level meter, in which the filters "A," "B," and "C" have been substituted by filters of different kinds. The rest of the instrument is essentially the same: The signal is detected by the microphone, filtered, processed, and then shown on the display.

There are several types of analyzers; however, here we will only deal with the types most commonly used: those equipped with 1/1 and 1/3 octave band filters. Because of the similarity between SLMs and analyzers, many SLMs allow the filters to be connected externally, so that the same instrument can perform both functions. The filter set can easily be attached to the SLM. Otherwise it is kept in the carrying case for when is needed.

The photograph in Figure 4–5 shows the Quest Model OB-300 filter set. It contains 1/3 octave band filters from 12.5 Hz to 20 kHz and 1/1 octave band filters from 16 Hz to 16,000 Hz. The photograph in Figure 4–6 shows a Quest Model 2900 sound analyzer comprising both an SLM and a filter set. This combination performs all the measurements that can be done by a SLM and by an analyzer.

To operate the analyzers described above, one has to click the octave (or the 1/3 octave) bands one by one, wait until the display stabilizes, and then read the sound level. Doing so requires that the sound level and the frequency content remain constant during the duration of the measurement and this often takes several minutes. Most noises demonstrate changes in both level and frequency, which make the measurement difficult and time consuming.

This problem has been solved by the so-called real time instruments, in which the signal is analyzed simultaneously by all filters and then integrated for a period of time determined by the operator (usually for 10 s). Each filter gets the same signal, solving the problem of signal variations. At the end of this period, the result is stored and displayed on the screen as a complete spectrum of the signal. Because the signal is processed several times at great speed, the displayed level is the average of all measurement results. An electronic pointer and a digital numeric display allow an exact reading of the sound level at a given frequency (i.e., one can move the pointer to a given frequency and the level at that particular frequency will be displayed).

Most analyzers have the possibility of storing the results of several measurements. Thus, for example, one can just walk around the floor

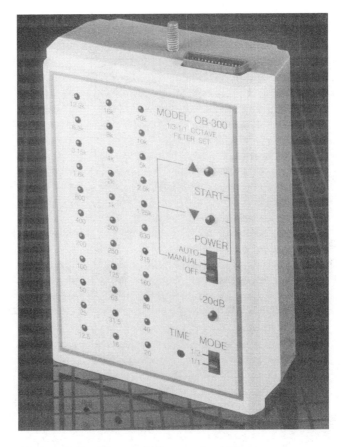

Figure 4–5. Octave and 1/3 octave band filter set.

of a factory, taking measurements at different locations. At the conclusion, all results can be either shown on the screen or sent as computer files to be further processed. Then the results can be printed out as a table or as a graph. Thus the time spent performing the actual measurements is minimized.

THE NOISE DOSIMETER

Occupational hearing loss results from exposure to high noise levels for long periods of time, day after day, year after year. There are very few occasions where the cochlea has been damaged instantaneously. Even when exposed to explosions or air blasts, damage is most often located in the external ear or the middle ear.

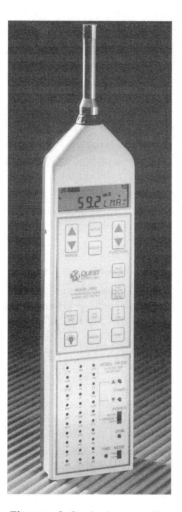

Figure 4–6. Analyzer resulting from a combination of a SLM and a filter set.

The use of a simple SLM is appropriate for the assessment of the hazard of a noise that is steady in nature. Since the level is constant, the display of the instrument allows for an accurate reading without fluctuations.

However, when a person is exposed to noise that varies in level and/or frequency content, a SLM cannot provide reliable results. This is a frequent situation in most occupations either because the sources are variable in their characteristics or because the person has to walk from one noisy location to the other. Thus an instrument capable of measuring the average noise level a person has been exposed to is required. The integrating SLM can perform that function. However, to do so, it has to be held close to the ear of the exposed person for the entire period of time. Obviously, this is not practical.

The solution is the noise dosimeter, an ISLM designed to be worn by the person whose noise exposure has to be measured. It is about the size of a pack of cigarettes (see Figure 4–7). The small microphone (1/8–in. diameter, covered with a windscreen in the picture) is connect-

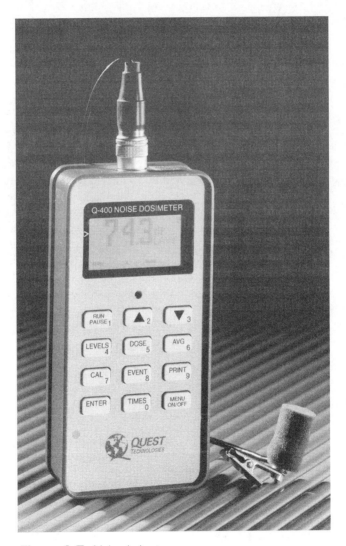

Figure 4–7. Noise dosimeter.

ed to the instrument's case through a long cable so that it can easily be attached to the wearer's shirt collar. The dosimeter itself is usually carried in the breast or pants pocket. Dosimeters' cases are sturdy, designed to stand the rough treatment on the plant floor. In many models the controls and the display can be covered by a metal lid, so that no part of the instrument is exposed.

Most dosimeters allow for the measurement of noise exposure using 3, 4, or 5 dB exchange rates.[3]

There are two types of dosimeters: the regular instruments and those that have a logging function. The regular instruments show on the display the final L_{eq} or L_{OSHA}. Some can also show the highest level reached during the measurement period as well as the duration period. Logging dosimeters are much more sophisticated instruments. They not only process the signals they detect, but they also store raw data for processing later in many different ways. At the end of the measuring period, they can calculate the L_{eq} or L_{OSHA} for different periods of time (e.g., 1 min, 1 hr, etc.) and generate a table with those values on a computer. They can also draw a graph showing the time distribution of the above-mentioned values. The time period they can measure is quite extensive: For example, they can measure the noise exposure of a person for 5 days, 8 hours/day, while logging the results.

Obviously, the logging dosimeter has many advantages compared to regular dosimeters. They are invaluable when one wants to determine which activity contributes by how much to the overall noise exposure of a person, a situation often found when someone does several different jobs during the workday. However, one has always to decide if the information obtained is really needed and if data that could be obtained using a regular instrument are not sufficient for the intended purpose. For example, if the purpose is just to assess if a person is overexposed, then the use of a regular instrument provides enough information and there is no need to use more sophisticated equipment.

NOISE EXPOSURE SURVEYS

Introduction

Noise exposure surveys are performed on individuals or on a group of workers. In either case there is a need for preliminary briefing of each

---

[3]The exchange rate is defined as the number of dB that a noise increases each time the exposure time is halved, to maintain the same exposure. When using the 3 dB exchange rate (adopted by NIOSH, ISO, and most of the provinces in Canada), the result is known as L_{eq}. When using the 5 dB exchange rate (used by the EPA and the Province of Ontario), the result is known as L_{OSHA}.

person who will be surveyed. He or she has to know why the measurement is needed, why he or she has been chosen, and should be given general information about the instrument itself. In other words the subject must be involved in the measurement as a willing partner for two important reasons:

1. This person will be using an instrument that costs in excess of $800.00 (U.S.). Although a sturdy instrument, it is still an electronic device that is not difficult to damage. If the wearer suspects that the result of the measurement will be used against him, or even if he was forced to wear it ("because I tell you to do so"), then there should be no surprise if the worker reports at the end of the shift that the dosimeter was accidentally dropped or the microphone cable was caught in a piece of machinery and chewed up, or any other real or imaginary damage. There have been several horror stories of instruments being intentionally damaged, because workers suspected that they were tape recorders used to eavesdrop on their conversations.

2. There is a natural tendency to show that the situation is worse than it is in reality. People who perform surveys are used to hearing from workers that the day they are surveying is actually a very quiet one with no noise at all compared what is normally the situation. Following this reasoning, it is not out of question to find the dosimeter left on top of a noisy machine or that the wearer shouts every so often into the microphone, to increase the measured noise exposure. Therefore, even if the instrument has not been damaged, the result of the measurement is faulty and inaccurate in such instances.

Noise Exposure Measurement on Individuals

The procedure for performing the measurement on an individual is relatively simple. It begins with the calibration of the instrument and the check of the batteries. Then the instrument is turned on and placed in the wearer's pocket with the microphone securely attached to his or her shirt or coat collar, close to the ear. Care should be taken that the microphone cable is not left loose and dangling, so that there is no hazard to the person or to the equipment. The person is then instructed to wear the dosimeter for the whole shift, including all breaks.

At this time the operator notes the calibration and the time the instrument was started. It is a good practice for the operator to take frequent noise level measurements close to the person wearing the dosimeter, so that he or she knows what to expect from the dosimeter reading at the end of the shift. Also, it is recommended that the activities performed by the wearer be logged.

At the end of the shift, the instrument's display is read, the batteries and calibration are checked again, and the results of the measurement are communicated and explained to the person who was wearing the dosimeter. The wearer must know what the result was. This builds trust between wearer and operator, so that in a similar situation, there will be no need to repeat lengthy explanations.

Noise Exposure of Groups[4]

The above procedure is used when the noise exposure of an individual is to be measured. However, it is impractical for a large number of workers, as it would require the use of one dosimeter per person. It also would require the analyst to work full time through many days to survey all of the workers in a plant. (Even more complex situations are found in the construction industry where tasks, as well as the work environment, are constantly changing.)

The solution is to measure the exposure of an entire group of workers by statistical methods. In this case, the group is treated as a population. A statistically significant sample of workers is measured and the results are processed so that they can be applied to the entire population. Then the noise exposure of each individual is expressed as a percentage of the probability that the noise exposure level will be below the safe level defined by the authority (85 dB or 90 dB), or as an average noise exposure level.

---

[4]The group is defined as workers performing the same activities or being in the same acoustical environment.

5

Hearing Protection Devices

earing protection devices were used first historically in the "high tech" fields such as the aircraft industry and later in a more general industrial "low tech" environment. The industrial usage initially resulted in a "one size fits all" philosophy regardless of input noise spectrum; however, as more became understood about hearing protection and its relationship to hearing in noise, the specifications became more appropriate.

Hearing protection devices should be considered for use in hearing conservation after other more global mechanisms for the reduction of noise exposure have been considered and implemented. In fact, in many hearing conservation laws, this relegation of hearing protection devices to a "last resort" is explicitly specified. Only after engineering controls and administrative controls have been implemented to their fullest to reduce the noise exposure of workers should their use in the work environment be considered. This means that reduction of noise at the source by repairing and/or muffling equipment, retrofitting with quieter equipment, treatment of the work area by erecting sound barriers or applying absorptive materials, turning off equipment while not in use, moving equipment away from the employees, or moving the employees away from noisy equipment, must have been explored and either ruled infeasible or implemented in a reasonable fashion.

The importance of reducing noise exposure levels in the work environment *before* assessing the need for hearing protection devices becomes apparent when the financial and personal costs of the use of hearing protection devices to prevent excessive noise exposure are considered. Financial costs of the use of hearing protection devices include, but are not restricted to:

- the provision, fitting, and replacement of the devices to employees
- provision of regularly-scheduled training programs for employees and supervisors in the correct use of the devices
- loss of productivity time while regular in-service training on hearing protection use occurs
- monitoring the correct use of the devices
- potential compensation claims if hearing loss is accrued despite hearing protection device use
- dealing with noncompliant employees who fail to regularly wear their hearing protection.

A review by Berger (1996) indicated that, in studies of workers in the United States and Canada published in the years 1990–1995, estimates of employees who usually wore their hearing protection devices all of the time ranged from a low of 5% (industrial arts teachers) to a high of 95% (police officers during firearm practice). In most cases, the compliance rate was between 30 and 60%.

Personal costs of the use of hearing protection may include:

- hearing loss if hearing protection provides insufficient protection or is improperly or inconsistently worn
- some workers will feel uncomfortable wearing their hearing protection
- some workers, particularly those with existing sensorineural hearing losses, may experience communication difficulties while wearing hearing protection
- allocation of responsibility for hearing protection from employers to employees

Thus, the use of hearing protection devices as part of a hearing conservation program involves more than the purchase and distribution of earplugs and earmuffs. To be successful, hearing protection devices should be part of an integrated, well-planned hearing conservation program.

OVERVIEW OF ATTENUATION CHARACTERISTICS

Hearing protection devices, whether they are earplugs or muffs, serve to protect the ear from excessive noise exposure by reducing the level of airborne sound that reaches the eardrum via the ear canal. However, hearing protection devices are limited in the amount of protection that they can provide. There are theoretical limits to the attenuation that can be produced in the ear by any earplug, earmuff, or other ear level hearing protection device.

To understand these theoretical limits, we must be cognizant of the multiple paths of sound transmission to the ear when an earplug or muff is worn. Sataloff (1993) has summarized these paths of sound transmission to the ear as four distinct, but related, sound paths. The first of these paths is the vibration of the bone and tissues of the skull and head. The second is a vibration of the hearing protection device itself while being worn. The third is leakage through the hearing protection device via porosities in the hearing protection device; these can be a function of the material of the hearing protection device, or of abuse and misuse of the hearing protection device. Finally, sound may enter the ear canal via leaks around the hearing protection device. Such leaks may occur when the hearing protection device is not used properly, is old and worn, or when the device has come loose during the day.

Many studies have examined the bases for the maximum attenuation levels from hearing protection at specific frequencies (Zwislocki, 1953, 1957; Shaw and Theissen, 1958, 1962; Berger, 1986). These factors pertain not only to the thickness and density of the material used in hearing protectors, but also to the level of bone-conducted sound transmission. Berger (1986), in reviewing the methods to assess the attenuation of hearing protectors, noted that at 2000 Hz, the bone conduction limit for hearing protection was the lowest (40 dB). That is, any measured attenuation greater than 40 dB in the 2000 Hz region represents artifacts of the "objective" measuring system. At this level, sound is conducted through the temporal bone directly to the cochlea, bypassing the air conduction route. One can measure an attenuation in excess of 40 dB at 2000 Hz by the use of artificial test fixtures (ATF) or by a real-ear-probe microphone measurement technique (such as microphone-in-real-ear [MIRE]), but these values would not correspond with subjective performance. The only exception would be the work of Schroeter (1986), where he constructed an ATF with as much inherent self-insertion loss as possible, and then accounted for the bone conduction route by post-measurement computational corrections. Figure 5–1, from Berger (1986), shows the bone conduction limits across frequency for hearing protector attenuation.

Closely related to this is the level of the occlusion effect. Discussed in more detail in Chapter 6, this effect is the improvement of the lower frequency bone conduction thresholds upon occlusion of the ear canal. This results in the amplification of internal physiological noise that masks the low-frequency unoccluded thresholds (Berger & Kerivan, 1983). The essential characteristics of this phenomenon were first delineated by Zwislocki in the 1950s (Zwislocki, 1953, 1957). Figure 5–2, from Berger (1988), shows how the occlusion effect varies with the volume of air enclosed between the hearing protector and the eardrum.

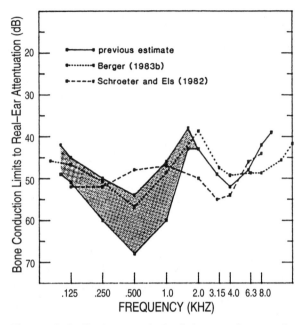

Figure 5-1. The bone conduction limits across frequency for hearing protector attenuation. The maximum attenuation at 2000 Hz is 40 dB. (From "Methods of measuring the attenuation of hearing protection devices," by E. H. Berger, 1986, *Journal of the Acoustical Society of America, 79,* 1655–1687. Reprinted by permission.)

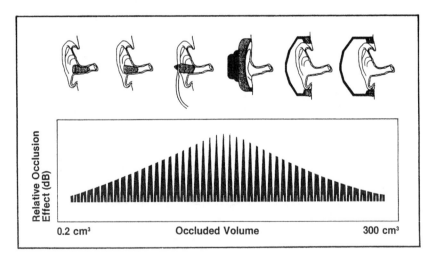

Figure 5-2. The occlusion effect varies with the volume of air enclosed between the ear protector and the eardrum. (From "Tips for fitting hearing protectors," by E. H. Berger, 1988, E•A•RLOG, 19. Indianapolis, IN: Cabot Safety Corporation. Reprinted by permission.)

The occlusion effect is well known in the hearing aid field and typically results in an echo-like sensation being reported by hearing aid users. Extension of the bore of the hearing aid canal into the bony portion of the external ear canal can reduce the occlusion effect. The extent of the occlusion effect can be measured clinically with the use of real-ear-measurement equipment as well as by hand-held occlusion effect meters.

Another feature of hearing protection is that, unless specifically designed otherwise, higher frequency sounds are attenuated more than the lower frequency sounds.

Figure 5–3 shows the frequency-dependent characteristics of a typical industrial foam plug deeply inserted into the ear canal. Two acoustic phenomena account for the frequency dependence and these have both been introduced and discussed in Chapter 3.

The first phenomenon is that all frequencies whose one-half wavelength is less than the diameter of the obstruction (or hearing protector) are attenuated. Low-frequency sounds (i.e., long wavelengths) are acoustically "myopic" and do not see the obstruction, but the shorter wavelength higher-frequency sounds acoustically see the obstruction. Although beyond the scope of this book to fully explain the physical issues, the effects of stiffness and mass also need to be considered. Nixon, Hille, and Kettler (1967) reported essentially no attenuation for the very low-frequency sounds (from 30 to 100 Hz).

The second phenomenon pertains to the existence of a quarter-wave resonator due to the presence of the ear canal. The human ear

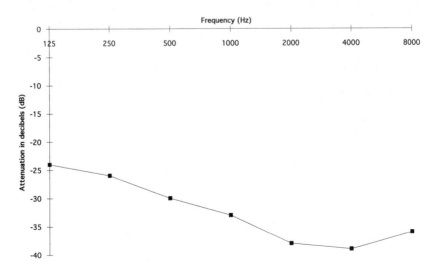

Figure 5–3. Attenuation characteristics of a typical industrial foam earplug that is deeply inserted into the ear canal. (From *Musicians and the Prevention of Hearing Loss* by M. Chasin, 1996. San Diego, CA: Singular Publishing Group.)

canal is on the order of 25 mm (one inch) in length that is closed at the tympanic membrane side and open at the lateral side. Such a tube behaves as a quarter-wavelength resonator with a frequency in the 2700 Hz region. The magnitude of the resonance is approximately 17 dB. This resonance is well known when dealing with hearing aids and is referred to as the *real ear unaided response* (REUR). Whenever the ear canal is occluded (with a hearing aid or a hearing protector), this naturally occurring resonance is lost. With earplugs, an additional high-frequency (insertion) loss is caused by this destruction of the 2700 Hz resonance.

In contrast, earmuffs do not destroy the natural ear resonance in the 2700 Hz region, and as such there is less relative high-frequency attenuation than if earplugs were used. Earmuffs do, however, yield greater attenuations in the 500–1000 Hz region. As an additional side effect, as can be observed in Figure 5–2, the level of the occlusion effect will be less with large volume earmuffs than with many earplug fittings.

One cannot, however, state definitively that the use of earmuffs yields improved intelligibility in noise over the use of earplugs, since hearing loss configuration and large subject variability are confounding factors (Abel, Alberti, Haythornwaite, & Riko, 1982).

Killion, DeVilbiss, and Stewart (1988) devised a custom earplug with approximately 15 decibels of attenuation over a wide range of frequencies. This was based on earlier work of Elmer Carlson. The earplug, named the ER-15 (manufactured by Etymotic Research, Inc.), has become widely accepted by musicians as well as by some industrial workers who work in relatively quiet environments. Figure 5–4 shows the attenuation characteristics of the ER-15 earplug along with the ER-25 earplug, the vented/tuned earplug, and an industrial-type foam plug for comparison purposes. Figure 5–5 shows the effect the ER-15 has on the spectrum of a violin (A_4 [440 Hz]) played at a mezzo forte level. Note that the attenuated spectrum is essentially parallel to the unattenuated one.

The design of the ER-15 earplug (and its partner, the ER-25 earplug that provides approximately 25 decibels of uniform attenuation) is remarkably simple. Essentially, a button-sized element that functions as an acoustic compliance is connected to a custom ear mold, with the volume of air in the sound bore acting as an acoustic mass. The resulting resonance between the compliance and the mass is in the 2700 Hz region and is designed to offset the insertion loss caused by the earplug. The high-frequency resonance is sufficiently broad to compensate for the relative high-frequency attenuation. Because the ER-element is manufactured in the factory, the compliance value is constant. Ear mold laboratories use a "mass meter" to verify that the custom ear mold has the correct volume of air in the sound bore in order to establish an essentially flat attenuation pattern. A schematic of the ER-15 is shown in Figure 5–6.

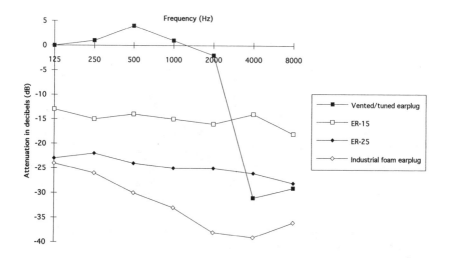

Figure 5–4. Attenuation characteristics of the ER-15, ER-25, and the vented/tuned earplugs. The industrial earplug data is also given for comparison purposes. (From "A clinically efficient hearing protection program for musicians," by M. Chasin and Chong, 1992, *Medical Problems of Performing Artists*, 7(2), 41. Adapted by permission.)

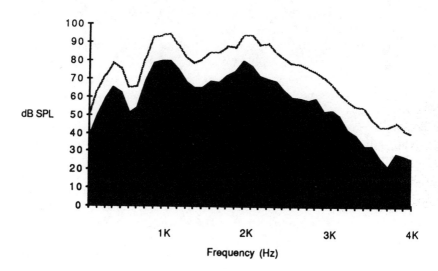

Figure 5–5. The effect of the ER-15 earplug on the spectrum of a violin playing the note A_4 (440 Hz). The attenuated spectrum (beneath) is parallel to the unattenuated one (above). (From "A clinically efficient hearing protection program for musicians," by M. Chasin and Chong, 1992, *Medical Problems of Performing Artists*, 7(2), 42. Reprinted by permission.)

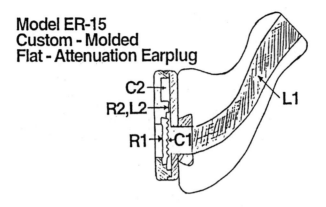

Model ER-15
Custom - Molded
Flat - Attenuation Earplug

Figure 5–6. A schematic of the ER-15 earplug. See text for explanation. (Courtesy of Etymotic Research.)

Because the ear mold is a custom-made product, the length of the sound bore can be made as long as possible. As pointed out by Zwislocki (1957) as well as is shown in Figure 5–2, the deeper the end of the ear mold in the ear canal, the less the occlusion effect. Research with completely-in-the-canal (CIC) hearing aids indicates that this can be clinically achieved if the mold terminates 2–3 mm inside of the bony portion of the ear canal (Chasin, 1994).

A noncustom (and less expensive) product is also available, called the ER-20/HI-FI earplug (Killion, Stewart, Falco, & Berger, 1992), and essentially uses the folded horn concept to enhance the higher frequencies and thereby reduce the high-frequency attenuation. The folded horn concept is a modification of the acoustic transformer effect discussed in Chapter 3, where the flaring tube is folded on itself because of space limitations but the high-frequency enhancement is maintained. This idea was used unsuccessfully in the mid 1980s to obtain some of the horn benefits for in-the-ear hearing aids (Gauthier & Burak, 1983). The other purpose of the folded horn is to relocate the sound entry point for the earplug from a position about 15 mm outside the entrance of the ear canal to the floor of the concha where there is significant high-frequency amplification.

Figure 5–7 shows the ER-20/HI-FI earplug. This earplug has a noise reduction rating (NRR) of 12 dB, and a new version with an NRR of 16 dB is also available. Unlike the ER-15 and ER-25 earplugs, the ER-20/HI-FI earplug has a slight high-frequency roll-off with attenuations ranging from 15 dB for the lower frequency sounds to 22 dB for the higher frequency sounds.

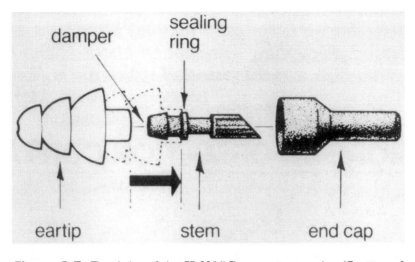

Figure 5-7. The design of the ER-20/HI-FI non-custom earplug. (Courtesy of Etymotic Research. A similar non-custom device called the NST is also available through Dalloz Safety.)

The ER-series of earplugs can be modified for those musicians with unusual ear canal resonances (not 2700 Hz) or for those with unusual hearing requirements, possibly due to a mild hearing loss.

In order to provide the theoretical basis for the clinical modification of the ER-series of earplugs, one can also view of the mass of air in the earplug sound bore as an inductance (*L*). The resonant frequency of this system can be given as being proportional to the square root of the inductance (*L*) over the compliance (*C*). *C* is a constant and is set by the design of the attenuator button. However, the inductance (*L*) is proportional to the length of the sound bore and inversely proportional to the cross-sectional area of the sound bore. The summarizing equation is shown in Figure 5–8.

TYPES OF HEARING PROTECTION DEVICES AND THEIR USE

In order for any hearing protector to attenuate sound across the broadest possible frequency range, the device must form an acoustic seal. Because individual ear canals differ in width, length, malleability, and shape, a single earplug or cap will not fit all persons equally well. The

$$FREQres \alpha \sqrt{L/C},$$

$$\text{where } L \alpha \text{ (length/cross-sectional area)}$$

Figure 5-8. The summarizing equation providing the theoretical basis for the clinical modification of ER-series earplugs.

fit of ear muffs can be affected by head size, jaw movement, and hair texture. Selection of appropriate hearing protection for a given employee will depend, therefore, on these individual factors as well as job-specific factors.

There are three primary types of protection devices: plugs, muffs, and ear caps. Each will be discussed below.

Plugs and Ear Caps

Ear caps are worn on the surface of the canal entrance and may enter only slightly into the canal. Caps are attached to a tension band that, depending on the type, may be worn over the head or under the chin. The pressure produced by the band on the cap forms the acoustic seal with the ear. Ear caps are easily donned and removed, and are very useful when temporary hearing protection is needed. However, ear caps typically do not provide as much hearing protection as muffs and plugs, and therefore may not provide adequate protection in some noise environments.

Earplugs form an acoustic seal within the ear canal. They can be made of a variety of products and may either be formable, taking their shape when placed in the ear canal, or custom formed, being made from an individualized ear canal impression. Formable plugs most commonly are made of dense foam, but may also be made of enclosed cotton, wax, or other malleable materials. Plugs made of rubber with a number of protruding flanges are also available (see Figure 5-7).

Many earplugs can be ordered with safety accessories attached to prevent the plugs from contaminating industrial materials should they inadvertently fall out on the job. For instance, plugs may have a neck cord attached to them, so that when removed they can be draped around the neck. Metallic nuggets can be included in the plug, so that the plugs can be detected should they fall into containers.

Both plugs and ear caps fit into the ear canal to block the path of sound to the ear drum. Prior to fitting either, the ear canal must be examined to ensure that there is not an excessive accumulation of wax (cerumen) that may be pushed further into the canal when the hearing protector is worn. Any lesions, growths, or other medical conditions in the canal contraindicate use of plugs until clearance by a physician is obtained. Caps may be worn if the problem in the canal is beyond the depth of the cap.

Customized earplugs can be obtained that are tailor-made for each individual's ears (Figure 5–6). They require that ear canal impressions are carefully and skillfully made by an experienced professional such as an audiologist or hearing aid dispenser. When fit properly, such plugs will provide long term comfort and hearing protection and need only be washed regularly to stay hygienic. Contact with perspiration and other agents will eventually cause deterioration of the ear mold material, making the plugs uncomfortable or ill fitting. Custom made plugs should also be refitted after a major weight loss or gain or any other time that a snug acoustic seal is not obtainable.

Insertion of foam plugs is best attempted in front of a mirror at first to gain some visibility of the ear and plug. The plug should be rolled gently between the thumb and the middle or forefinger until it is compressed (Figure 5–9a). Gently pull the earlobe back and slightly upwards (Figure 5–9b). For most people, this will open and straighten the ear canal (and is best observed by examining the effect on another person's ear). Insert the compressed plug into the ear canal, until the outside end of the plug is flush with the end of the ear canal. Keep the fingertip over the end of the plug for about 15 seconds to allow the compressed plug to expand in the canal and to prevent it from expanding out of the canal. A correctly sized and positioned earplug should feel snug in the ear canal, and should not protrude into the bowl (concha) of the ear. Figure 5–9c shows a well-positioned plug and Figure 5–9d shows a plug that is providing only minimal attenuation because it is occluding only a small portion of the ear canal.

Three simple tests can be used to establish whether an earplug has formed an acoustic seal properly (Royster & Royster, 1994). The "tug test" is suitable for plugs with removal handles or neck cords. A gentle tug back and forth on the handle should cause a mild sensation of suction in the canal or on the eardrum when the plug has formed a good seal. The "hum test" can be used when a single plug has been inserted. When the wearer hums, the voice should sound louder in the adequately plugged ear, because of the occlusion effect discussed above. When the second plug is inserted, the voice should appear equally loud in both

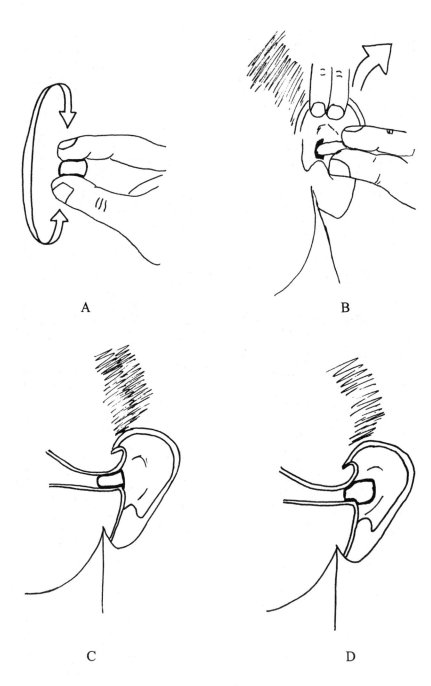

A

B

C

D

Figure 5–9. Insertion of formable foam earplugs.

ears. Finally, the "loudness test" can be used in a noisy environment. When a person is wearing well-fitted plugs in noise and cups both hands over the ears, the perceived noise level should not change. When the seal of the plug is broken, the noise level should be heard to increase.

Although most formable plugs can be reused several times and remain effective, they will lose their capacity to expand completely in the ear canal with repeated use and should be replaced as directed by the manufacturer. For employees in many jobs, daily replacement of formable plugs may be desirable because perspiration, dust, chemicals, or other agents may render the plugs unsanitary after a single use.

Formable plugs, custom-made earplugs, and other devices that are seated in or on the ear, may need to be reseated during the day. Movement of the jaw while talking, speaking, or chewing gum may loosen a plug in the ear canal, and force it slightly out of the ear canal, so that the attenuation provided by the plug is reduced. Frequent monitoring of the hearing protection device will ensure that the device continues to provide sound attenuation throughout the day. Ear muffs may loosen or be pushed askew, reducing their effectiveness.

Ear Muffs

Ear muffs fit over the ear and form an acoustic seal around the ear. The attenuation provided by the muff is a function of the materials contained in the muff, and the adequacy of its acoustic seal. The band of the ear muff is therefore an important factor in maintaining the integrity of the ear muff; pressure provided by the band should be sufficient to completely seal the ear. Attempts to loosen the headband to improve comfort may decrease the sound attenuation provided by the ear muff.

Ear muffs can be made compatible with a wide assortment of other safety equipment, including safety helmets, goggles, hoods, and visors. Extreme care should be taken, however, when combining these safety devices, so that they do not interfere with each other's function or create a hazard themselves (for instance, by reducing the wearer's field of vision). Table 5–1 compares comfort, hygiene, safety and cost factors for different types of hearing protectors.

Whether the employee chooses to wear plugs, caps, or muffs, or a combination of plugs and muffs, adequate and continuing education needs to be provided along with the hearing protection device. A hearing protector will take time to become part of the work routine, may be felt as a distraction when initially worn by the employee, and will require some personal adjustment. Employee questions and concerns about using hearing protection need to be answered on an ongoing basis, not just once during the initial introduction of the devices.

TABLE 5-1. Comparison of hearing protection devices.

Considerations	Custom Plugs	Disposable Plugs	Muffs	Canal Caps
Insertion	easy to insert after initial learning period	takes care and instruction	easy to slip on and off	easy to slip on and off
Hygiene	may get dirty w/ handling generally easy to clean	may get dirty w/ handling	easy to clean	may get dirty w/ handling but can be held by band to keep caps cleaner
Comfort	after initial adjustment period - excellent	after initial adjustment period - good	hot, sweaty, headband pressure may bother some	after initial adjustment period - good
Safety	may be difficult to retrieve from equipment - small size	may be difficult to retrieve from equipment - small size	may be integrated with other equipment (hard hat; visor)	band under chin may interfere with other equipment
Daily Maintenance	cleaning and drying	not required	wipe clean	wipe clean
Anticipated length of use	1-2 years	1-3 days	6 mos - 2 yrs	months
Cost per unit (2 ears)	$100 and up	$0.60 and up	$15 and up	$1.50 and up
Visibility	low	low	high	moderate
Susceptibility to ineffective use (inadequate protection)	low	high	moderate	high

Changes in what is heard by the employee may require some re-learning of equipment sounds and may produce an often unjustified concern that communication is impaired when the hearing protectors are worn.

Thus employees must be provided with ongoing support for the fitting, adjustment, and replacement of the hearing protectors, and also for any adjustments and concerns that they may have while using the devices.

ELECTRONIC BASED HEARING PROTECTION

Several innovations have allowed some forms of hearing protection to be based on electronic characteristics rather than acoustic ones. The first innovation was *active noise reduction* (ANR) and is based on the principle that two identical signals, when added together out of phase, will cancel. While it is difficult to assess a quickly varying signal and generate another with the identical spectrum but 180° out of phase, it is a relatively easy task for steady state signals, especially if they are low frequency (i.e., long wavelength). ANR hearing protection has not gained wide acceptance because of its high cost, its limitation to low-frequency attenuation, and up until recently, its limitation to relatively steady state signals (Figure 5–10).

In contrast, *active sound transmission* hearing protection has had its major use in hunting where optimal hearing of the movement of the prey has to be coupled with optimal hearing protection. A modified hearing aid circuit is typically utilized that allows for amplification at low input levels but attenuation or clipping at higher levels (such as the blast from a gun) (Figure 5–11). An external monitoring microphone is used to assess the environmental noise/music level, and the amplification stages are reduced or disabled completely above a certain preselected level. Electronically based hearing protection of this type has been used for percussion musicians but typically only during practice sessions.

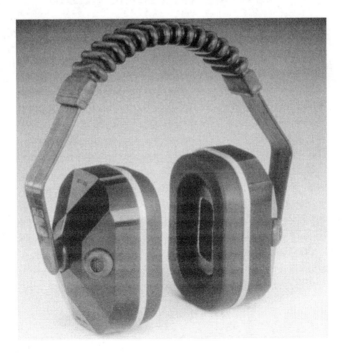

Figure 5-10. An Active Noise Reduction headset, using phase cancellation. (Photograph courtesy of E.A.R.)

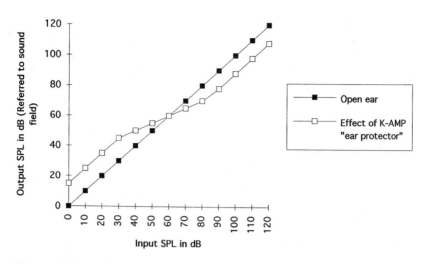

Figure 5-11. Input/output curve for a hearing aid with a K-AMP circuit showing amplification for lower input levels and attenuation for higher input levels. (Courtesy of Etymotic Research.)

ASSESSMENT TECHNIQUES

There are several objective assessment techniques to determine the attenuation of hearing protectors. Berger (1986) pointed out that the term "attenuation" is rather poorly defined and that instead there should be a discussion of insertion loss and noise reduction.

Insertion loss is a similar measure to insertion gain in the hearing aid field in that two consecutive measures are made with miniature microphones. Insertion loss can be assessed objectively using a microphone-in-real-ear (MIRE) technique. Such a technique is analogous to the real-ear-insertion-response (REIR) for hearing aid assessment. One measure is made in the ear canal without the hearing protection and the other is made in the identical location with the hearing protection in place. The difference is the insertion loss. Because the location of the microphone is identical in both conditions, all factors that affect the SPL, other than the decrease in SPL caused by the hearing protector, are subtracted. This measure is further discussed in Chapter 6 and tends to be the most expeditious for clinical use. A potential problem with the insertion loss measure is the inadvertent contribution of the bone conduction route.

Noise reduction is a simultaneous measure made by two separate microphones: one being outside of the hearing protector and the other being on the medial side in the ear canal. A noise reduction measure can be affected by the precise location of the microphone in the ear canal as well as by diffraction effects from the external portion of the ear canal.

Yet this measure can be useful in high noise environments and can utilize an actual industrial spectrum as the stimulus.

Subjective techniques can be categorized as *threshold-based,* or *supra threshold.* Threshold-based techniques are the oldest and in most cases provide a high degree of reliability. Associated with any subjective technique, the individual's ability to respond is a factor and this contributes an inevitable source of error. For this reason, the standard deviations tend to be higher than for those techniques that utilize an objective microphone-based procedure.

Real ear attenuation at threshold (REAT) is a subjective technique that seeks to assess the change in the hearing threshold of a subject with and without hearing protection. REAT can be assessed under earphones or (binaurally) in the sound field. Two drawbacks of this measure (especially if measured in the sound field) are an inability to attain a quiet enough environment to achieve a true unprotected condition, and low-frequency masking may occur as a result of physiological noise that overstates the degree of low-frequency attenuation. When REAT is assessed under earphones, the first factor is rarely an issue, but corrections need to be made for a slightly smaller volume, as part or all of the concha is occupied by the hearing protector.

Suprathreshold-based techniques tend to have a poorer test-retest reliability than REAT and are not commonly used. These may include measures of midline lateralization, speech reception thresholds, and other psychophysical tests. For an excellent review of these techniques, the interested reader is referred to Alberti (1982) and to Berger (1986).

SINGLE-VALUE ATTENUATION RATING SCHEMES

Several single-number rating schemes are in use throughout the world. The most commonly used scheme in the United States is the Noise Reduction Rating (NRR). Most parts of Europe use an octave band method as well as the ISO recommended Single Number Rating (SNR) (E.H. Berger, personal communication, 1995). Most provinces in Canada use the ABC scheme where hearing protectors are categorized according to a standard (Z94.2–94) into Class A, B, or C depending on their octave band attenuation values and the measured L_{eq}Na time weighted average (Behar & Desormeaux, 1994).

The NRR has been in widespread use since 1979 as a relatively simple method to characterize the attenuation of hearing protectors. The NRR innovation came from the work of Botsford (1973), who found that the environmental noise measured in dBC (dB C-weighted) and the noise level measured in dBA (dB A-weighted), when assessed in the ear canal with the hearing protector in place, was a constant and could be used to characterize the hearing protector (Figure 5–12).

However, as pointed out by Preves and Pehringer (1983), the NRR calculation made some simplifying assumptions and required the use of various correction factors. The validity of these assumptions has led to some criticism of the NRR technique. One such assumption is that the environmental noise spectrum is a constant pink noise, having equal octave band levels across the spectrum.

To understand the potential problem with this assumption, it may be useful to review and compare the C-weighting and A-weighting networks. The C-weighting network is essentially no weighting at all—less than a 1-decibel effect up to 6000 Hz. However, the A-weighting network attempts to simulate human hearing sensitivity—a significant low-frequency roll-off of up to 16 decibels at 125 Hz, with no effect at and above 1000 Hz. Thus, if an environmental noise spectrum has significant low-frequency energy, the dBC measure will be much greater than the dBA measure. In contrast, if there is minimal low-frequency noise, there will be minimal difference between a dBA and a dBC noise measurement.

When a comparison is made between a C-weighted measurement and an A-weighted one, a preliminary form of spectral analysis is being performed. Clearly, accepting the NRR without reference to the spectral shape of the environmental noise can be a major source of error.

The work of NIOSH (see Chapter 2) yielded a correction factor of 3 dB in the calculation of the NRR because some workers do not wear their hearing protection properly, as well as for reasons pertaining to the spectral uncertainties just mentioned. Johnson and Nixon (1974) felt that this correction factor should be 5 or 6 dB. As this figure would be subtracted from the calculation, the NRR would be a worst case scenario. The NRR for each hearing protector is a measure based on the results of a number of subjects. Subsequently a two standard deviation pad is also included as "a statistical adjustment so that the mean values are modified to reflect what some larger proportion of the population will actually achieve" (E.H. Berger, personal communication, 1995). This two standard deviation range covers approximately 95% of the population. The NRR formula is given in Figure 5–12.

As can be seen, if the true noise spectrum has no low-frequency energy (as it may be with treble musical instruments), then the first two terms are identical, and the NRR is simply the attenuation and associated wearing and statistical factors. For the musician's ER-15™ uniform attenuator earplug, the octave band attenuation is approximately 15 decibels, with the calculated NRR being only 7 dB. Johnson and Nixon (1974) noted that the NRR tends to be artificially high if there is minimal low-frequency attenuation and would be artificially low if there was a flat attenuation characteristic.

The American Speech-Language-Hearing Association has stated that the NRR is "an inadequate predictor of 'real' hearing protector

NRR = N (C-weighted) - N (A-weighted) + attenuation (A-weighted) - 3 dB - 2 standard deviations

Figure 5-12. The formula for the calculation of the Noise Reduction Rating (NRR).

effectiveness" (1997, p. 34) and is searching for more suitable alternative methods.

Although simplifying measures such as the NRR have made hearing protector characterization easier for the laboratories, the NRR tends to be affected by many artifacts when used for a different purpose than originally intended. It is, unfortunately, a widely held view that the higher the NRR, the better the hearing protector. Depending on the noise or music level, the spectral shape, and the individual's communication or musical requirements, this is certainly not the case. Killion (1993) summarized this with a current day fallacy: *Parvum bonum, plus melius,* which means "A little is good: More is better."

SUMMARY

Hearing protectors, unless specifically designed, attenuate the higher frequency sound energy more than lower frequency energy. Because such a nonuniform attenuation characteristic can be less than optimal for certain high-fidelity requirements, acoustically tuned hearing protectors were developed. Such earplugs can be used in the performing arts and in industrial settings with noise levels below 100 dBA.

Objective techniques such as microphone-in-real-ear (MIRE) and the use of acoustical test fixtures (ATF), and subjective techniques such as REAT, are two valid methods for assessing the effects of hearing protection. Regardless of the technique, the resulting data can be expressed in a single-number rating scheme such as the Noise Reduction Rating (NRR), but caution should be taken in fitting hearing protection on the basis of such a single-number rating unless the parameters of the industrial noise match those used in generating the rating value. Constant vigilance must be maintained by employees and supervisors to ensure that hearing protectors are always worn properly in high noise environment on the job site.

Noise Control

As described in previous chapters, noise can cause several undesirable effects such as hearing loss, annoyance, work interference, and so on. These all affect humans and, occasionally, animals. However, noise as such is not a problem, unless someone is or will suffer some effects from noise.

WHY AND WHEN SHOULD
THE NOISE BE CONTROLLED

When thinking about noise control, there are a couple of questions to be asked before attempting any action. The first question is: Who is affected? If there is no one who could suffer some effects from noise, then there is no need for action and for investing any resources.

The second question is: If the noise is affecting people, and some control has to be instituted, by how much must the noise level be reduced? For example, if we are dealing with annoyance in a rural area, then the noise levels should, most probably, have to be reduced down to some 40 or 50 dBA. If, on the contrary, the issue is occupational noise in a factory, then the upper limit for the noise level will be 85 dBA. Therefore, just mentioning that the noise has to be controlled is not sufficient: The maximum allowable level has to be known. To find the answer to that question, one has to refer to local municipal laws, and existing state, federal, or provincial legislation. Only then, by knowing the existing level and the allowable limit, will one know how much the noise level has to be reduced.

From there on, the control process takes place: The frequency analysis of the noise must be performed, the way in which the noise reaches the receivers has to be determined, and, finally, the proper noise control measure has to be implemented.

In summary, the two questions that have to be answered before any noise control project is instituted are:

1. Is anyone affected by the noise?
2. By how many decibels must the noise be reduced?

At the end of the process, the cost also has to be estimated. In the case of occupational noise, there are situations where it is not feasible or economical to institute engineering noise controls and hearing protectors must be used.

If the problem is office noise or environmental noise, obviously the use of protectors is out of the question and noise has to be reduced by other means, one of which could be the relocation of the noise source. There is no unique answer or solution to the problem. Each situation has to be examined separately before attempting any noise control solution.

THE BASIC APPROACH: SOURCE, PATH, RECEIVER

When dealing with noise control, the following three basic issues have to be addressed:

1. The source of the noise (e.g., a machine, a factory, a highway),
2. The path, or the way the sound is transmitted from the source to the receiver (through the air or the ground), and
3. The receiver (e.g., a worker or a neighbor).

The task of the noise engineer is to properly identify each of these elements and to know their characteristics. Because each of them can theoretically be controlled, the decision of which way to go is taken only after carefully considering the feasibility and the cost associated with each approach.

The need to determine the source is obvious. Its noise characteristics, sound level, frequency distribution, and directionality pattern have to be known. Usually, they can be obtained from the manufacturer or through measurements.

The path the energy is following from the source to the receiver must be clearly identified. Failure to do so may result in the use of a wrong control. For example, if the motor of an elevator is transmitting vibrations to the floor, and the result is noise perceived several floors below the motor room, increasing the room insulation will not solve the problem. The proper way to go will be to insulate the vibrations transmitted from the motor to its base, so that the vibration path is interrupted. Only then will the noise decrease or disappear.

The same principle applies to the noise generated by the ground vibrations of the tracks due to the passing of a train, on the surface or underground. Unless the tracks are properly isolated,[1] the noise will continue to be generated because of the ground vibrations.

However, if a properly isolated compressor generates high airborne noise levels, then this is the path that has to be controlled, using either noise barriers or enclosures.

Another issue that has to be examined is the presence of other sound sources in the vicinity. The noise generated by the second source or by the environment, in the case of outdoor noise control, is also known as *background noise*. It marks the lowest limit for noise reduction. There is no point in reducing the noise of a source below this level, since there will be no perceived or measured improvement in a given situation.

For instance, if a noise source is generating 90 dBA on a factory floor, there obviously is no point in reducing the noise level of other sources to below this level.

In another situation, if we are dealing with the installation of a cooling tower that may affect a neighbor, the noise generated by a nearby highway may be a limiting factor for the noise level limit requested by the authorities. If the regulation asks for a maximum level of 45 dBA and the highway is generating 55 dBA, then the noise control project should aim at a level that will not elevate the 55 dBA noise floor. As discussed in previous chapters, if the new noise source (the cooling tower, in this case) generates a noise level of 47 dBA at the neighbors' premises, the noise resulting from the combined effect of the highway and the tower (47 + 55 dBA) will not exceed significantly the existing 55 dBA. (Of course, attention should be given to other issues, such as wind direction, weather conditions, day and night operation, etc.)

NOISE SOURCE

As mentioned above, the characteristics of the noise source have to be known as a first step in a noise control project. Among those characteristics the most important is, without any doubt, the frequency spectrum. In most occasions, the octave band analysis between the frequencies of 125 and 8000 Hz is sufficient. Sometimes, although not too often, there is a need for narrow band analysis, as is the case when the design of a pure tone silencer is needed.

The directivity factor of a noise source is another characteristic that may be needed, especially when dealing with outdoor sources. It provides information about how much of the acoustical energy flows in a

---

[1] The term "insulation" is applied to sound, while "isolation" is used for vibrations.

given direction. This information is especially useful when dealing with outdoor sources.

If the directivity factor is supplied by the manufacturer of the noise source, and if it is possible to do so, the source should be oriented so that the disturbance is minimal. There have been occasions in which simply reorienting the source solved the problem. An example for such a procedure is found when dealing with large electric power transformers, where sound radiates preferably from the front and the back of the transformer and much less from the sides. By choosing a proper orientation, noise levels at the receiver site can be substantially reduced.

If the source is already installed, not much can be done, except to attempt to rotate the source so that the radiation is minimal in the direction of the affected neighbor.

SOUND PROPAGATION: AIRBORNE AND STRUCTURE-BORNE, INDOOR AND OUTDOOR

Airborne and Structure-Borne

In most situations, noise is transmitted through the air. The vibrating object (or its parts) that are in contact with the air generate an oscillatory motion that propagates, maintaining the same vibrating characteristics (mainly the frequency) of the source. This applies to most of the noise-generation phenomena, such as:

- Normally vibrating sources (vibrators, shakers, conveyers),
- Impact noise sources (hammers, presses, riveters, office printers), and
- Gases/liquids flow noise sources (flow in ducts, exhausts, valves).

However, there are situations where the source communicates vibrations to its base. Such vibrations, if not controlled, propagate freely through the entire structure. As a result, noise can appear far away from the source as the result of the vibrations of a wall, or the floor.

Structure-borne and airborne noise are controlled using different materials and procedures. What is good for one is worthless for the other. Therefore the exact determination of how noise propagates from the source to the receiver is of utmost importance.

In this chapter, we will be dealing basically with airborne noise, occasionally mentioning some situations when the structure-borne path is of importance.

Sound Propagation Indoors

If the noise source is contained within a room, once generated, the noise energy travels from the source to the limiting surfaces (ceiling, walls, and floor). While travelling, there is certain reduction of the noise energy, due to the sound absorption through the air and also because of the dispersion from the area of the source to the entire volume of the enclosure. If the dimensions of the site are not too large, the noise level reduction with the distance from the source is of very little importance.

Once the energy has reached the limiting surfaces, then, as explained in Chapter 1, part is reflected and part is transmitted through the walls to the other premises or outside of the locations. The amount of reflected energy depends on the acoustical properties of the limiting surfaces: The more absorbent they are, less energy is reflected, and, therefore, the resulting noise level will be lower.

Most industrial sites are characterized by having acoustically "hard" surfaces. There is almost no absorption in metal-clad walls, a cement floor, and metal sheet ceilings. Therefore, the noise travels back and forth, reflected by the surfaces, with little attenuation. The net result is that the sound level is almost the same close or far away from the source.

This kind of environment is known as *reverberant*. If an impulse noise is generated in such an environment, it persists for a long time and the resulting noise level is slowly reduced. The same phenomenon occurs in most non-acoustically-treated spaces such as churches, swimming pools, assembly halls, and so on. Besides having high noise levels, speech intelligibility in these sites is very poor unless specific electro-acoustic measures are implemented.

The control of those situations is further examined in the section on noise absorption.

Sound Propagation Outdoors

When sound travels outdoors, its energy decreases with distance and the sound level is reduced by 6 dB every time the distance is doubled. For instance, if the noise from a plant is 60 dB at 100 m, it will be 54 dB at 200 m and 48 dB at 400 m. This rule is an approximation that does not take into account the environmental conditions, nor the sound reflection from the ground, but it still can be used as a guideline for sound reduction with distance.

This situation is approximated in enclosures with highly absorbent limiting surfaces (e.g., inside of a recording studio or in an anechoic chamber), where the conditions of propagation become closer to this in the open and the noise level decreases as the distance from the source increases.

NOISE CONTROL AT THE SOURCE

The most efficient way of controlling noise is at the design stage. This principle applies not only to noise sources, but also to industrial plants and office/residential buildings. As with illumination, ventilation, piping, and so on, noise sources, their location, and insulation should be studied, so that when the place is ready for occupation, there is no need for costly and often inefficient retrofittings.

In the case of an existing noise source, retrofitting requires in-depth knowledge of the machine/device, knowledge that only the manufacturer possesses. Therefore, getting "inside" is an almost forbidden action that may also imply the end of the manufacturers' warranty, as is stated in most documents.

Lately, in most situations, source control is done by the manufacturer, as it is in the manufacturer's interest to deliver a product as user friendly as possible. This trend has been enhanced in the European Common Market, where machines must be labeled with their noise output, thus giving the purchaser the option of acquiring quieter machines. Although in the USA and Canada there is no legislation that requires labeling, exporters who deal with the European market have to also label their products. That is why they are already in the process of reducing their noise output.

There are situations in which a simple modification of peripheral devices may reduce the noise significantly. This, for example, is the case with the exhaust of compressors and compressed air valves, drivers, and cleaners. A simple silencer attached to the exhaust reduces the air turbulence without adding a significant load to the exhausting air. On the other hand, using silencers without going through the appropriate studies may increase the back pressure and adversely modify a process.

All of the above suggestions refer to new equipment. However, much is to be said with respect to the increase of the noise with age and improper maintenance. Here is a short list of steps that can be easily performed and will reduce significantly the noise emission of equipment already in use:

1. Periodic balancing of rotating parts. It is well known that improper balance leads to vibrations, increases noise levels, and reduces equipment life.
2. Proper lubrication of moving parts is also a factor in noise reduction. Old or inappropriate oil increases the noise of ball bearings. Use of the right cutting oil is essential for reducing the cutting noise associate with machining.
3. If there is an acoustical enclosure, it should be properly maintained and used as required.

NOISE CONTROL OF THE PATH

Once the possibility of controlling the noise at the source has been exhausted, the next stage is to try to eliminate or reduce the transmission of the noise energy from the source to the receiver.

To begin with, the path followed by the noise (or the structure-borne vibrations) has to be thoroughly determined. Structure-borne vibrations tend to be quite complex and require specific materials for their control. Fortunately, in most situations, noise is transmitted through the air. This is the reason for limiting our scope to the airborne transmitted noise only.

Two different situations may arise:

1. If we are dealing with external noise, then the solution of choice is the use of barriers. This is the case with highway noise, as well as with cooling towers, roof-mounted air conditioning units, truck loading docks, and so on.
2. If both the source and the receiver are inside the same building, then an acoustical enclosure has to be used for either the source or the receiver to block the passage of the acoustical energy.

Both barriers and enclosures have to block energy. To do so they have to be built using specific materials and procedures. Acoustical insulation, which is how the procedure is known, will be dealt with later in this chapter.

Acoustical Barriers

Acoustical (noise) barriers act as partial enclosures by interrupting the direct flow of noise energy from the source toward the receiver. The phenomenon is similar to throwing an acoustical shadow toward the receiver. If sound energy propagates in a straight line, then it will go from the source to the barrier, will be reflected, and no energy will reach the receiver, leaving it completely isolated. This is what happens with light when an obstacle is placed between the source and the receiver. However, as discussed in Chapter 1, the sound "shade" is not complete because part of the energy is refracted from the edges of the barrier (upper and lateral). This is especially true at lower frequencies (below 500 Hz), when the wavelengths of the noise are comparable to the size of the barrier.

In addition to frequency dependence, the barrier effectiveness is related to its height and the distances to the source and to the receiver: The higher the barrier and the closer the distances, the better the protection offered by the barrier.

There are practical limitations to the height. For structural reasons it seldom exceeds 6 m. Because the wind load increases with height, the barrier will require expensive supportive structure and the cost will proportionally increase. There are also esthetic reasons for avoiding very tall barriers.

The barrier also cannot always be located close to the source. For instance, highway noise barriers cannot be placed closer than the right of way, which greatly reduces their effectiveness for the noise originated from the traffic lane opposite to the barrier. A similar situation of distance limitation appears when erecting a barrier close to a water cooling tower: Because of the ventilation, the barrier cannot be too close to the tower.

Another issue in considering the barrier choice for noise control is its length. Since noise is diffracted not only from the top but also from the edges of the barrier, the barrier has to be longer than the source. In practice, barrier length is designed to be equal to the length of the noise source (or receiver) plus one height of the barrier on each side.

The effectiveness of a barrier is defined in terms of *insertion loss* (IL), defined as the difference between the noise level at a particular location without and with the barrier in place. IL can be expressed in dBA or in octave bands. IL is always much higher at high frequencies. However, the practical limit that can be achieved at any given frequency is 20 dB.

Barriers can also be used inside a plant. In that case, care should be taken to reduce the energy reflected by the ceiling, as it will add to the diffracted energy, and thus reduce the barrier's effectiveness.

Acoustical Enclosures

An enclosure is similar to a barrier, with the difference that the enclosure completely cuts the flow of the energy to the surrounding space. Because of the total surrounding, there are no refraction phenomena. The only way the acoustical energy can escape or penetrate an enclosure is through the enclosure's limiting surfaces: walls, ceiling, and floor, or through the openings: doors, windows, and conduits.

The concept of duality is valid in this case: The acoustical energy is the same whether "escaping" or "penetrating" an enclosure; therefore the design for noise control is the same in both cases. The only difference is that when dealing with enclosures for the receiver (the worker) other ergonomic issues, such as ventilation, illumination, accesses (both physical and visual), and so on, must be considered.

ACOUSTICAL INSULATION

Transmission Loss (TL) and Sound Transmission Class (STC)

As mentioned before, the scope of this section is limited to air transmitted sound. This by no means implies that the structure-borne sound should be neglected. As discussed above, knowledge of the sound path is of utmost importance for effective noise control. However, structure-borne noise is not found as often as airborne noise.

The sound insulation of a partition is measured and defined in terms of transmission loss as follows:

$TL = 10 \log L_{tr} / L_{in}$ (dB)
where L_{tr} is the energy transmitted through the partition, and
L_{in} is the incident energy, which reaches the partition.

The measurement of TL is done in specially designed laboratory facilities, where two rooms ("transmission rooms") are joined by an opening where the partition that is to be measured is located. Several loudspeakers generate the test signal in one of the rooms (transmitting room), while the measuring microphones installed in both rooms measure the sound level in the transmitting room and in the receiving ("quiet") one. The measurement is performed following national and international standards at 125, 250, 500, 1000, 2000 and 4000 Hz. The TL is calculated using the difference between both sound levels, corrected by the characteristics of the receiving room. The larger the TL, the better the sound insulation. Most building materials have been measured and the resulting TL can be found elsewhere. When using those TLs, it has to be remembered that they are results from laboratory measurements and that the values found in the field are often reduced because of poor workmanship, openings, and so on.

Results of the measurements are shown in tables, as Table 6–1, where TL is represented as a function of the test frequency.

TL is seldom used for qualifying a material, or a partition, because of the difficulty in dealing with several numbers, one for each test frequency. Instead, the Sound Transmission Class (STC) is the characteristic most often being reported. STC is a single number, which is obtained through calculations using the TL results. As with TL, the larger the STC, the better the acoustical insulation offered by a partition.

Transmission loss and sound transmission class are both characteristics of a given material or an infinite partition. In practice, noise reduction is affected by the quality of workmanship, the presence of windows

TABLE 6–1. Transmission Losses of Some Materials (dB)

	Frequency, Hz						
Material	*125*	*250*	*500*	*1000*	*2000*	*4000*	*8000*
Steel, 18-gauge	15	19	31	32	35	48	53
Plywood, 3/4" thick	24	22	27	28	25	27	35
Plexiglass, 1" thick	25	28	32	32	34	46	46
Glass, 1/4" thick	17	23	25	27	28	29	53
Concrete, 4" thick	29	35	37	43	44	50	53
Brick, 4" thick	30	36	37	37	37	43	—
Single wood stud wall	20	36	39	46	42	53	—

and doors, and also by the amount of sound absorbing materials in the quiet side of the partition. For that reason, there is another characteristic that is being measured: the noise reduction (NR), also expressed in dB. As with the other sound insulating characteristics, NR is also dependent on the test frequency. NR is defined as follows:

$$NR = TL + 10 \log \alpha/S \text{ (dB)}$$
where α is the total absorption in the receiving (quiet) room, and S is the surface of the wall transmitting the noise (the wall between both rooms).

The above expression shows that, for a given transmission loss, the sound level in the receiving room will decrease if more sound absorption is installed. Sound absorption is dealt with in the next section.

To sum up, the best noise reduction is obtained by using partitions with high TL and by using sound absorption in the room that is designed to be quiet.

Sound Insulation from a Single Partition: the Mass Law

The simplest partition is the single partition, consisting of single layer of sound insulating materials. A brick wall, a dry wall, and metal cladding of an industrial building are all examples of single wall partitions; they are often used because of their low cost and ease of construction. However, there are still problems, related mainly to the workmanship, that must be properly resolved to obtain best results. For example, the

TL of a brick wall will greatly decrease if the mortar is applied in a sloppy way, leaving holes between the bricks and a door that is not properly adjusted will offer an easy pathway for acoustical energy through the resulting opening.

TL of a single partition can be calculated using the so called Weight-Mass Law, an empirical rule, which states that the TL of a single partition increases up to 6 dB per doubling of the frequency and also 6 dB per doubling of the surface weight.

The mathematical expression of the law is:

TL = 14.5 log m + 14.5 log f - 26 dB.
where   m is the surface weight in kg/m^2, [2] and
           f is the frequency

Figure 6–1 shows a graphic representation of the Mass Law for the frequency of 500 Hz. It can be seen that the TL of a partition with a surface density of 100 kg/m^2 is 42 dB at 500 Hz. At 1000 Hz it will be 6 dB higher (48 dB).

Sound Insulation From a Multiple Layer Partition

The drywall used typically as a partition between two rooms in a house is constructed using two panels separated by airspace. The use of this type of construction increases the TL in the following way: If the distance between the two layers is quite large (e.g., larger than 50 cm), then both partitions will act independently, and the total TL will be equal to twice the individual TLs.

If the distance between them is zero then, according to the Mass Law, the total TL will be equal to the individual one, plus 6 dB, resulting from the doubling of the mass.

In most practical situations, we are dealing with distances of up to 25 cm for walls or up to 12.5 cm for window panes. In those cases, the resulting TL is higher than predicted by the Mass Law but still lower than the sum of both TLs. The exact values cannot be predicted theoretically and we have to rely on data obtained through laboratory measurements.

TL of a multiple layer partition can be improved significantly by filling the cavity between the partitions with sound absorbing materials (e.g., fiberglass or polyurethane foam).

---

[2]Surface weight of a material or partition is defined as the density of the material, in kg/m^3 multiplied by its thickness in meters.

Sound Insulation From Composite Partition

In many situations we have to deal with partitions made from different parts. The best example is a wall that has a window and/or a door.

The calculation of the TL from such a construction is quite complex. However, the rule of thumb is that the resulting TL is closer to the TL of the material that is the poorer insulator. For example, if a wall is made of bricks and has a door that is lightweight, with a hollow core, the resulting TL will be similar to that of the door and the insulation of the wall will be wasted because of the poor TL of the door.

By the same token, if a partition has an opening, the resulting TL will be drastically reduced. This, for example, might be the case of the window in the wall between the dispatcher's room and the loading dock in a warehouse. Even if the wall between them has a large TL, if the window is just an opening in the wall (as it is in most cases), the resulting TL will be low enough as to significantly elevate the noise in the dispatcher's room.

SOUND ABSORPTION

Sound Absorption and the
Noise Reduction Coefficient (NRC)

Sound absorption is a physical phenomenon by which sound waves that impinge on a surface lose some of their energy while being reflected back to where they came from. In summary, we may say that sound insulation is related to a sound wave passing through a partition, whereas sound absorption is related to a wave remaining in the same site. By the same token, sound insulation deals with noise emerging from an enclosure, while sound absorption deals with noise that remains inside the enclosure.

Sound absorption is measured in laboratories using specific facilities called reverberant rooms or an acoustic instrument known as the Kundt tube. Absorption is measured in Sabine, which is equivalent to the sound absorption of an open window with a surface area of 1 m². Thus the largest absorption coefficient that can be obtained has the value of 1 Sabine.

Although they are completely different phenomena, sound absorption and sound insulation have some similarity. As with the sound insulation, sound absorption varies with frequency. For most sound-absorbing materials, the absorption is low at low frequencies and increases as the frequency rises. In the same way as with the sound insulation, absorption is measured at 125, 250, 500, 1000, 2000, and 4000 Hz. For the same rea-

Mass Law
Transmission Loss, dB (500Hz)

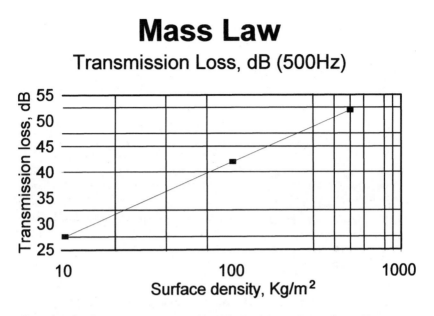

Figure 6–1. Graphic representation of the Mass Law for the frequency of 500 Hz.

sons as with the STC, the noise reduction coefficient (NRC) has been introduced as a single number descriptor of the absorption quality of a material. It is defined as the arithmetic average (the mean value) of the absorption at 250, 500, 1000, and 2000 Hz.

Echo, Reverberation, and Sound Absorption

A well known phenomenon, the echo, consists in perceiving a sound reflected from a large surface (wall, hill, wood) as distinct from the original. Generally it is generated using short duration, impulse sounds, such as clapping hands, a gunshot, or a scream. Shortly after the sound has been emitted, it "comes" back as if emitted from the obstacle. If there are several reflecting surfaces, far away from each other, as is sometimes the case with deep ravines, several echos may be perceived for each sound being emitted.

To be perceived as distinct, the reflected signal has to arrive with at least 0.1 second delay.[3] To do so, the obstacle has to be at a distance of

---

[3]The 0.1 second is the minimum time needed by the brain to recognize the two signals as distinct.

some 15 m or more from the source. If the delay is shorter, the sensation is that the signal has been extended—its time duration is longer and the sound level sounds louder.

If there is more than one reflecting surface close to one another (e.g., in large auditoriums, gymnasiums, churches, etc.), there will be multiple reflected sounds arriving at different times, all with a very short delay. The perceived sound is then of a single sound that persists for a long time, with a sound level that is slowly decaying.

This is a phenomenon called *reverberation*. There is also a specific term: "reverberation time," which is the time that takes for the sound level to decay 60 dB from its initial level. Because the speed of the decay of the level depends of the amount of energy that has been absorbed after each reflection, the reverberation time is strongly related to the total sound absorption in an enclosure.

This relation is as follows:

$$RT = 0.16 \, V/A$$
Where RT is the reverberation time in seconds,
     V is the volume of the room in m^3, and
     A is the total sound absorption of the room in Sabine.

The RT is a useful quantity when measuring the sound absorption of a material in the reverberation room mentioned above. For that purpose, RT is measured before and after introducing the material in the room. The difference between the two RTs at each frequency is used for the calculation of A.

The correct reverberation time is very important when dealing with acoustics of rooms used for speech and/or music. If RT is too short, then the hall sounds "dead." If it is too long, it sounds too "alive" and the intelligibility is poor. Depending on the size and the use of the place, the optimum RT has been specified and can be found elsewhere in the literature. To adjust the RT of a hall to the optimum value, sound-absorbing materials such as carpets, curtains, drapes, and so on, are introduced. Because of the strong relation between the sound absorption coefficient and frequency, special absorbing devices are needed to ensure the optimum RT is achieved at all frequencies.

Sound Absorption and Noise Control

In an enclosure, the sound level is the complex result of the direct and all reflected sounds. As explained above, the reflected sounds are reduced by using high sound absorption on the limiting surfaces. However, no sound absorbing treatment can reduce the direct sound.

That is why the use of sound absorption for noise control purposes is limited to situations where the receiver is not too close to the source.

Table 6–2 shows the sound absorption of some common materials and also of some acoustical materials. The unit here is percent. To obtain the value of sound absorption in Sabine, this percentage has to be multiplied by the surface that has been used. In other word, a small surface covered with a highly absorbent material is the same as a large surface with a material with a low sound-absorbing coefficient.

A general formula for noise reduction in dB, by using sound absorption is:

$$NR = 10 \log A_2/A_1$$

where A_2 is the total absorption in the room in Sabine after the treatment, and

A_1 is the total absorption in the room in Sabine before the treatment.

To illustrate the power of the use of sound-absorbing materials, it has to be said that the maximum theoretical noise reduction is of some 15 dB. However, in practice, it rarely exceeds 7–10 dB. It all depends on the distance of the receiver with respect to the source: The shorter the distance is, less effective is the treatment. On the other hand, a small difference may be all that is needed to eliminate the hazard in a workplace.

The application in which sound absorption is most important is when dealing with speech intelligibility. The use of sound-absorbing material can change dramatically the sound or speech quality of a hall, increasing the ease of communication.

TABLE 6–2. Sound Absorption Coefficients of Some Materials

	Frequency, Hz					
Material	**125**	**250**	**500**	**1000**	**2000**	**4000**
Acoustic tiles, fiberglass	0.63	0.9	0.68	0.9	0.96	0.91
Theater audience	0.52	0.68	0.85	0.97	0.93	0.85
Heavy carpet	0.08	0.24	0.57	0.69	0.71	0.73
Concrete blocks, unpainted	0.36	0.44	0.31	0.29	0.39	0.25
Cork, 1" thick	0.25	0.55	0.7	0.75	0.75	0.75
Curtains, light	0.03	0.04	0.11	0.17	0.24	0.35
Window glass	0.35	0.25	0.18	0.12	0.07	0.04
Plaster	0.14	0.1	0.08	0.05	0.04	0.03
Water (surface of pool)	0.01	0.01	0.01	0.015	0.02	0.03

Sound Absorption Materials and Devices

The term "acoustical material" is extensively used, although, as we know now, materials can be either absorbing or insulating. No material can fulfill both functions, since good insulators are bad absorbers and viceversa. Therefore, simply mentioning this term can be misleading: it has always to be specified what kind of materials or properties one has in mind.

Insulating materials are heavy and must be airtight. Examples are building materials (bricks, gyprock, drywall), metal sheets, and glass.

Sound-absorbing materials, on the contrary, are light and porous. Examples are fiberglass, mineral wool, drapes, and seat covers. Some commercial materials are also available in the shape of acoustic tiles, wall coverings, or hanging panels. They all fall under the category of the so called porous absorbers, because the sound absorption is the result of the penetration of the acoustical wave into the pores of the material and the consequent transformation of the acoustical energy into heat. All porous materials exhibit low sound absorption at low frequencies and high at the other extreme of the frequency range. Figure 6–2 shows a typical curve of the sound absorption for this kind of materials.

On some occasions, however, there is a need for high absorption at the lower end of the spectrum. This occurs mostly when adjusting the reverberation time of an auditorium (also known as "tuning" the hall). In this situation, a porous absorber would not be the best choice and the so-called panel absorbers will have to be used. They will provide higher absorption at low frequencies and low at high. Panel absorbers are a special type of absorber that responds to different principles.

Another type of absorbers, used when dealing with narrow band frequency noise, are the Helmholtz resonators. Their absorption is limited to a relatively narrow band of frequencies, and they can be tuned to the frequency of the offending noise. Because of their limited use, they cannot be obtained off the shelf and have to be specifically constructed.

ABSORPTION OF A POROUS MATERIAL

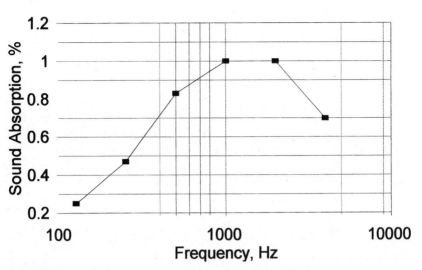

Figure 6-2. Typical curve of the sound absorption of a porous material.

7

Occupational Hearing Conservation Regulations and Standards

hroughout the United States and Canada, legislation has been enacted to restrict the amount of sound to which industrial[1] workers may be exposed. These hearing conservation laws represent the results of many compromises. These compromises are primarily the desire to protect workers' hearing health, to minimize the costs of doing business, and to enact enforceable legislation. The hearing conservation legislation adopted in each jurisdiction differs greatly, as a result of the compromises reached in individual constituencies. Hearing conservation regulations should *not* be viewed, therefore, as a means for defining "safe" exposure levels, that is levels at which exposed persons will not accrue a noise-induced hearing loss,[2] tinnitus, or nonauditory noise-induced disease. Rather, they describe levels that must not be exceeded in order to be in compliance with occupational safety regulations.

Some hearing conservation legislation is extremely brief, providing only an indication of the limits of noise levels to which employees may be exposed, whereas other legislation is detailed, and provides a relatively complete description of the required elements of a hearing con-

---

[1]The term "industrial" is ill-defined in many jurisdictions and may exclude a large number of employees. Persons employed in some fields who may operate in noisy environments, such as musicians, dentists, and hospitality workers, may not be covered by some industrial hearing conservation laws.

[2]It is not uncommon for people to use existing legislation to describe what is a "safe" noise exposure. In general, absolutely "safe" noise exposure levels are well below the limits specified in North American hearing conservation laws.

servation program. Comprehensive hearing conservation legislation contains not only precise definitions of such elements as exposure limits, but also specifies other aspects of hearing conservation, including, but not limited to, who is responsible for implementing hearing programs, who is involved in the audiometric testing of employees, when testing must be conducted, the specifics of any hearing protection devices to be used, the educational programs that must be provided, and the types and extent of any engineering controls that must be implemented.

In this chapter, a summary of the key points in hearing conservation legislation will be provided. Caution should be taken by all readers, however; these summaries, while providing a means of quantifying some elements of the diverse regulations cannot represent the details of the laws, legislation, and statutes. These summaries are provided, therefore, with the assumption that readers will consult the original legislative documents for their own jurisdiction and ensure that such legislation has not been replaced or amended.

To be useful to both employers and employees and to be enforceable, hearing conservation legislation must specify the measures that are needed in order to establish (1) whether noise exposure levels are exceeded by employees and (2) if so, what steps must be taken, and by whom, to reduce the noise exposure of employees. Furthermore, the legislation must specify how these measures are to be made, either explicitly in the legislation, or by reference to existing standards of measurement, as discussed later in this chapter. While the terminology used to denote these measures may differ in the various jurisdictions, the essential elements do not. The terminology provided in this chapter is consistent with common usage across much of North American hearing conservation legislation.

PERMISSIBLE EXPOSURE LEVEL

The permissible exposure level (PEL) is the maximum noise exposure level, generally measured in A-weighted sound pressure level (dBA) to which an employee may be exposed for a specific duration. In order to be specified completely, the PEL should include the sound level, including the units of measurement (usually dBA), the required parameters of the measurement device (such as crest factor, integration time, frequency response), and the duration of the noise exposure. In the United States and Canada, an 8-hour duration is specified for the daily exposure, with the assumption that this 8-hour period is representative of a common work shift.

Most industrial noise levels are not static and fluctuate throughout the exposure interval. Furthermore, exposure to noises greater than that indicated by the PEL may be allowable under some circumstances. As a result, other parameters of the sound exposure levels and duration of exposures need to be measured.

EXCHANGE RATE

The exchange rate defines the rate at which sound exposure levels may change with a concomitant change in the permissible exposure duration. Common exchange rates used in North America are the 3-dB and 5-dB per doubling rates. With the 3-dB exchange rate, for example, a 3 dB increase (or decrease) in exposure level will result in a halving (or doubling) of the duration that an employee may be exposed to such a noise. Thus, in a jurisdiction with a PEL of 90 dBA and an exchange rate of 3 dB, an employee may be exposed to a maximum of 90 dBA for an 8-hour shift; if the noise level is 93 dBA the employee may only work 4 hours in the noise before exceeding the permitted noise exposure limits.

Many noise measurement specifications report a *minimum sound level* that must be included in the exposure measures. This level is not specified by all regulations, but when specified, is frequently in the region of 70 to 80 dBA. Noise exposures below this minimum level need not be measured and are not included in the calculation of an employee's noise exposure or dose.

A maximum exposure level should also be specified. This is the noise level (in dBA) above which an employee must not be exposed without hearing protection, no matter how brief the exposure duration. This maximum level, when specified, is frequently 140 dBA. When this maximum level is left unspecified in noise legislation, the legislation is seriously flawed; theoretically an employee could be exposed to a level that could create immediate and permanent hearing damage, as long the duration of the exposure was sufficiently brief.

LEGISLATION IN THE UNITED STATES

In the United States, hearing conservation legislation is a federal mandate. The Occupational Health and Safety Administration (OSHA, 1983) noise standard covers employees in general and maritime industries (Suter, 1996). OSHA provides a comprehensive set of regulations for industrial hearing conservation, including noise exposure measurement, hearing conservation programs, monitoring, audiometric testing, hearing protection devices, employee training, record keeping, information access, and employee notification.

OSHA regulations limit the permissible exposure level for 8 hours to 90 dBA, with an exchange rate of 5 dB per halving of exposure duration, up to a maximum of 115 dBA. A percent noise exposure or noise dose, which represents a percentage of the maximum allowable noise exposure dose, can be computed using the tables provided in the OSHA legislation or using equation 7–1.

$$D = 100(C_1/T_1 + C_2/T_2 + ... + C_n/T_n), \quad (7–1)$$

where C_n is the exposure duration at a specific level and T_n is the maximum allowable duration at that level, as computed from equation 7–2.

$$T = \frac{8}{2^{(L-90)/5}} \quad (7–2)$$

where L is the A-weighted sound pressure level.

The time-weighted average (TWA) is a decibel-like measure that is the A-weighted "average" sound pressure level for an 8-hour day, when the averaging process uses the 5 dB exchange rate. TWA can be computed from the noise dose using equation 7–3.

$$TWA = 16.61 \log_{10}(D/10) + 90, \quad (7–3)$$

where D is the percent noise dose.

The maximum permissible dose is 100%, which is equivalent to an 8-hour TWA of 90 dB. When employees are exposed to levels that exceed this limit, administrative or engineering controls must be implemented where feasible. Administrative controls are methods that alter the employees' assignments to reduce the time spent in noisy situations. They may include such means as job sharing or job rotation. Engineering controls are methods that reduce the noise exposure by decreasing the amount of noise reaching the employee by means such as acoustic isolation or absorption, modification of equipment, or replacement of equipment with less noisy devices.

Employees who receive a TWA of 85 dB or greater, equivalent to a noise dose of 50% or more, exceed the action level. Noise monitoring must then be completed to determine which employees to include in a hearing conservation program. Any employees exposed to a TWA of 85 dB or greater must be notified of the results of the monitoring and an audiometric testing program must be established.

Audiometric testing programs consist of three parts (1) baseline audiogram, (2) annual audiogram, and (3) audiogram evaluation and follow-up. A baseline audiogram must normally be obtained within 6 months of a employee's first exposure at or above the 85-dB action level. The baseline audiogram is used as a basis for comparison for future audiograms. Audiograms must be obtained annually for all employees exposed to the action level or higher. Finally, an audiologist, otolaryngologist, or physician must review the annual audiogram, determine whether further evaluation is needed, and identify whether a standard threshold shift (shift or 10 dB or more at 2, 3, and 4 kHz) has occurred. Notification of the employee and assessment of hearing conservation measures are required when a standard threshold shift is detected.

Records of noise exposure levels and both baseline and annual audiograms must be maintained and made available to employees.

In addition to annual audiometric testing, all employees exposed at the action level or higher, must be provided with hearing protection devices as part of the personal protective equipment. A hearing conservation training program must be provided and information and training materials must be available to all affected employees.

Mine employees may be covered by the Mining Safety and Health Administration (MSHA) regulations for occupational noise exposure. MSHA currently allows a TWA of 90 dBA for 8 hours, with a 5-dB exchange rate. The maximum exposure level is 115 dBA. Discussions are currently underway to revise the MSHA standards for occupational noise exposure in coal, metal, and nonmetal mines. The proposed changes include the addition of an action level of 85 dBA, a minimum level of 80 dBA to be included in dose calculations, and the inclusion of a hearing conservation program, which consists of hearing testing. Mines may be covered by both MSHA and OSHA regulations.

Table 7–1 summarizes key limits specified by the OSHA and MSHA legislation.

The U.S. Air Force and Army have developed their own noise exposure guidelines to protect their employees' hearing. They limit the permissible exposure level to 85 dBA and use a 3-dB exchange rate to compute noise exposures (Suter, 1996).

LEGISLATION IN CANADA

In Canada, hearing conservation legislation is both a federal and provincial concern. Federal government employees and employees of certain industries that cross interprovincial boundaries fall under the jurisdiction of the federal legislation. The relevant federal legislation consists of three parts: the description of who is covered by the legislation, a section applicable to the interprovincial trucking industry (which has exposure limits based on those used in the United States), and a section for all other industries. Each province in Canada has its own hearing conservation regulations for employees not covered by the federal legislation. The permissible exposure levels, exchange rates, and requirement for audiologic monitoring of noise-exposed employees differ among provincial statutes, as does the level of detail provided by the statutes. Table 7–2 provides a summary of some of the limits defined by provincial and federal statutes.

TABLE 7-1. Summary table of occupational noise legislation in the United States

Jurisdiction	Minimum Level (dBA)	Maximum Allowable Level (dBA)	Action Level	Permissible Exposure Level (dBA)	Exchange Rate (dBA)	Maximum Peak Level (SPL)	Impulses (impacts) per Day	Audiometric Testing Required
OSHA	80	115	TWA of 85 dB or dose >50%	90	5	unspecified	unspecified	yes
MSHA[a]	80	115		90	5			no

[a] A set of MSHA proposed rule revisions has been prepared and changes are under discussion. Readers should consult the MSHA web page at http://www.msha.gov/regs for current information.

TABLE 7-2. Summary table of occupational noise legislation in Canada

Jurisdiction	Minimum Level (dBA)	Maximum Allowable Level (dBA)	Action Level	Permissible Exposure Level (dBA)	Exchange Rate (dBA)	Maximum Peak Level (SPL)	Impulses (impacts) per Day	Audiometric Testing Required
Federal[a] General	74	unspecified	84	97	3	unspecified	unspecified	no
Large trucks (1) (>4500 kg)		115		90	5	unspecified	unspecified	no
Alberta[b]	80	115	85	85	5	140	100@140 dB	yes
British Columbia[c]	≤80		82	85	3	135	not specified	yes
Manitoba[d]		unspecified	80	90	3	unspecified	unspecified	yes
New Brunswick[e]	80	115	80	85	5	140	100@140 dB	no
Newfoundland[f]			80	85	5	140	100	no
Northwest Territories[g]			90	90	5	140	unspecified	no
Nova Scotia[h]								
Ontario[i]		115	90	90	5	unspecified	unspecified	no
Prince Edward Island[j]		115	80	85	5	140	100@140 dB	yes
Quebec[k]		115	85	90	5	140	100@140 dB	yes (in some instances)

(continued)

TABLE 7-2. (continued)

Jurisdiction	Minimum Level (dBA)	Maximum Allowable Level (dBA)	Action Level	Permissible Exposure Level (dBA)	Exchange Rate (dBA)	Maximum Peak Level (SPL)	Impulses (impacts) per Day	Audiometric Testing Required
Saskatchewan[l]	80	unspecified	80	85	3	unspecified	unspecified	yes
Yukon[m]			80	85	3	140	90@140 dB	yes

[a]Canada—Federal jurisdictions: Canada Labour Code, Canadian Occupational Safety and Health Regulation, Part VII Levels of Sounds. http://canada.justice.gc.ca/cgi-bin/folioisa.dll/eregs.nfo

[b]Alberta: Alberta Occupational Health and Safety Act, Noise Regulation. http://www.gov.ab.ca/~lab/msbe/msb-e01.html

[c]British Columbia: Occupational Health and Safety Regulation, Part 7: Noise, vibration, radiation and temperature.

[d]Manitoba: Workplace Safety and Health Act, Hearing Conservation and Noise Control Regulation. http://www.gov.mb.ca/labour/safety/act/mr227-1.html

[e]New Brunswick: General Regulation: Occupational Health and Safety Act, Part V Noise, sec. 29-33; Hearing Protective Equipment, sec. 48.

[f]Newfoundland: Occupational Health and Safety Regulations, sec. 50; 58.

[g]Northwest Territories: Occupational Health and Safety Human Resource Material Section 1502: Protective clothing and safety equipment. Exposure limits are based on the ACGIH guidelines. http://www.gov.nt.ca/Publications/HR_Manual/1502.htm

[h]Nova Scotia: Occupational Health and Safety Act. Exposure limits are based on the ACGIH guidelines.

[i]Ontario: Ontario Industrial Establishments under the Occupational Health and Safety Act, sec. 139; Oil and Gas Offshore Regulations, sec. 41.

[j]Prince Edward Island: Occupational Health and Safety Regulations, Part 8.

[k]Quebec: Construction Safety Code, sec. 2.10.7; Regulation Respecting the Quality of the Work Environment, Division VIII: Noise.

[l]Saskatchewan: Occupational Health and Safety Regulation, 1996, Part VIII: Noise and Hearing Conservation, sec. 7.1-7.23.

[m]Yukon: O.I.C. 1986/164 Occupational Health and Safety Act. http://132.204.132.167/

WORKER'S COMPENSATION

Worker's compensation for occupationally induced hearing loss is provided through state worker's compensation legislation in the United States[3] and by provincial compensation boards in Canada. The criteria for determining a compensable hearing loss are not consistent across these jurisdictions. For insured employees, audiologists, and other hearing health care professionals, extreme care must be taken to ensure that any documentation of noise-induced hearing losses will meet the requirements of the worker's compensation law in their region. For example, many compensation laws require information about hearing thresholds at 3000 Hz, a frequency that may not be tested in some routine audiometric evaluations. Many laws also include "corrections for age," which are adjustments to measured hearing levels that reflect the expected decline of hearing thresholds of the worker based on advancing age.

ACOUSTICAL STANDARDS
AND STANDARD ORGANIZATIONS

A standard is a document that sets a value that has been approved by consent. There are measurement standards that describe the instruments that must be used, their characteristics, the way the measurements must be performed and, finally, how results must be presented.

Other standards deal with instruments, describing their characteristics and accuracy, for example. Finally, there are standards that must deal with devices, such as hearing protectors, describing how they must be measured and how they must perform.

Standards are written by experts in their own fields. In most cases, they are handled by nongovernmental organizations. Examples of such organizations are the American National Standards Institute (ANSI) in the United States and the Canadian Standard Association (CSA) in Canada. On the international scheme, there are two organizations—the International Organization for Standardization (ISO) and the International Electrotechnical Association (IEC), that write international standards. Presently, there is a growing tendency in countries to adopt international standards, something that makes a lot of sense, because the specialists who write the international standards are also members of the national standards organizations.

Following are the organizations whose standards are quoted here and also the list of those standards that are of interest to the readers.

[3]Cudworth (1986) provides a summary of compensation laws for U.S. states.

Standards Writing Organizations

ISO—International Organization for Standardization
Case Postale 56.
CH - 1211 Geneve 20, Switzerland
http://www.iso.ch

IEC—International Electrotechnical Commission
Rue de Varembe,
Geneve, Switzerland
http://www.iec.ch

ANSI—American National Standards Institution
120 Wall Street, 32nd Floor
New York, NY 10005 - 3993
http://www.ansi.org

CSA—Canadian Standard Association
178 Rexdale Boulevard
Toronto, ON Canada M9W 1R3
http://www.csa-international.org

Standards

ISO

ISO 1999–1990: Acoustics—Determination of occupational noise exposure and
    estimation of noise-induced hearing impairment
ISO 389 (Parts 1 through 7): Acoustics—Reference zero for the calibration of
    audiometric equipment
ISO 4869 (Parts 1 through 7): Acoustics—Hearing protectors
ISO 6189: 1983: Acoustics—Pure tone air conduction threshold audiometry for
    hearing conservation purposes.
ISO 7028: 1984: Acoustics—Threshold of hearing by air conduction as a function
    of age and sex for otologically normal persons.
ISO 31-7.1992: Quanitities and units—Part 7: Acoustics
ISO 266.1997: Preferred frequencies
ISO 8253 (1 through 3): Acoustics—audiometric test methods

IEC

IEC 651: Sound level meters
IEC 804: Integrating-averaging sound level meters
IEC 942: Sound calibrators
IEC 1252: Electroacoustics—Specifications for personal sound exposure meters

ANSI - ISO - IEC Catalog

ANSI - ISO-IEC Catalog: IEC 61252: Electroacoustics—Specifications for personal sound exposure meters
ANSI - ISO-IEC Catalog: IEC 61260: Octave band and fractional-octave band filters
ANSI - ISO-IEC Catalog: IEC 60942: Sound calibrators

ANSI

ANSI S1.1-1994: Acoustical terminology
BSR S3.20-1995: Bioacoustical terminology
ANSI S1.4-1983 (R1997): Specification for sound level meters
ANSI S1.4a-1985 (R1997): Amendment to ANSI S1.4 - 1983.
ANSI S1.9-1996: Instruments for the measurement of sound intensity
ANSI S1.25-1991 (R1997): Specification for personal noise dosimeters
ANSI S1.43-1997: Specification for integrating-averaging sound level meters
ANSI S3.6-1996: Specification for audiometers
ANSI S3.44-1996: Determination of occupational noise exposure and estimation of noise-induced hearing impairment
ANSI S12.6-1997: Methods for measuring the real-ear attenuation of hearing protectors
ANSI S12.13-1991: Evaluating the effectiveness of hearing conservation programs (draft)
ANSI S12.19-1996: Measurement of occupational noise exposure
ANSI S12.42-1995: Microphone-in-real-ear and acoustic test fixture methods for the measurement of insertion loss of hearing protection devices

CSA

CSA Z107.51: Procedure for in-situ measurement of noise from industrial equipment
CSA Z107.56: Procedure for the measurement of occupational noise exposure
CSA Z107.4: Pure tone air conduction audiometers for hearing conservation and for screening
CSA Z94.2: Hearing protectors

BIBLIOGRAPHY

American Conference of Governmental Industrial Hygiene. *Threshold Limit Values and Biological Exposure Indices.* (updated yearly).
CCH Canadian Limited (1999). *Canadian Employment Safety and Health Guide.* Don Mills, ON: CCH Canadian.
Feldman, A. S. and Grimes, C. T. (1985). *Hearing Conservation in Industry.* Baltimore: Williams and Wilkins.

Cudworth, A. L. (1986). Worker's compensation. In E. H. Berger , W. D. Ward, J. C. Morrill, and L. H. Royster (Eds.), *Noise and Hearing Conservation Manual.* Fairfax, VA: American Industrial Hygiene Association.

Health and Welfare Canada (1987). *Guideline for regulatory control of occupational noise exposure and hearing conservation: Part 1 - Model regulation.* Author.

OSHA (1981). Occupational Noise Exposure: Hearing Conservation Amendment. *Federal Register 46:* 4078–4179.

OSHA (1983). Occupational Noise Exposure; Hearing Conservation Amendment; Final Rule. *Federal Register 48:* 9738–9785.

Suter, A. H. (1996). Current standards for occupational exposure to noise. In A. Axelsson, H. Borchgrevink, R. P. Hamernik, P. A. Hellstrom, D. Henderson, and R. J. Salvi (Eds.), *Scientific Basis of Noise-Induced Hearing Loss.* New York: Thieme.

References

Abel, S. M., Alberti, P. A., Haythornwaite, C., & Riko, K. (1982). Speech intelligibility in noise with and without ear protectors. In P. W. Alberti (Ed.), *Personal hearing protection in industry*. (pp. 371–386). New York: Raven Press.

Alberti, P. W. (Ed.). (1982). *Personal hearing protection in industry*. New York: Raven Press.

American Conference of Governmental Industrial Hygiene. *Threshold limit values and biological exposure indices*. [updated yearly].

American Speech-Language-Hearing Association. (1997). Issues: Occupational and environmental hearing conservation. *Asha, 39*(Suppl.17), 30–34.

Bachem, A. (1955). Absolute pitch. *Journal of the Acoustical Society of America, 27*, 1180–1185.

Barone, J. A., Peters, J. M., Garabrant, D. H., Bernstein, L., & Krebsbach, R. (1987). Smoking as a risk factor in noise-induced hearing loss. *Journal of Occupational Medicine, 29*, 741–745.

Barrs, D., Althoff, L., Krueger, W., & Olsson, J. (1994). Work-related, noise-induced hearing loss: Evaluation including evoked potential audiometry. *Otolaryngology—Head and Neck Surgery, 110*(2), 177–184.

Baughn, W. L. (1973). *Relation between daily noise exposure and hearing loss as based on the evaluation of 6835 industrial noise exposure cases*. Aerospace Medical Research Laboratory, Wright-Patterson Air Force Base, Dayton, Ohio, TR AMRL-TR-73-53 (AD 767 204).

Behar, A., & Desormeaux, J. (1994). NRR, ABC or . . . . *Canadian Acoustics, 22*(1), 27–30.

Berger, E. H. (1986). Methods of measuring the attenuation of hearing protection devices. *Journal of the Acoustical Society of America, 79*, 1655–1687.

Berger, E. H. (1988). Tips for fitting hearing protectors. *E·A·RLOG 19*. Indianapolis, IN: Cabot Safety Corporation.

Berger, E. H. (1996). Industrial activities in the use, standardization, and regulation of hearing protection. *Journal of the Acoustical Society of America, 99*, 2463.

Berger, E. H., & Kerivan, J. E. (1983). Influence of physiological noise and the occlusion effect on the measurement of real-ear attenuation at threshold. *Journal of the Acoustical Society of America, 74*, 81–94.

Berger, E. H., Royster, L. H., & Thomas, W. G. (1978). Presumed noise-induced permanent threshold shift resulting from exposure to an A-weighted Leq of 89 dB. *Journal of the Acoustical Society of America, 64,* 192–197.

Berlin, C. I. (1994). When outer hair cells fail, use correct circuitry to simulate their function. *Hearing Journal, 47*(4), 43.

Bies, D. A. (1994). An alternative model for combining noise and age-induced hearing loss. *Journal of the Acoustical Society of America, 95,* 563–565.

Bies, D. A., & Hansen, C. H. (1990). An alternative mathematical description of the relationship between noise exposure and hearing loss. *Journal of the Acoustical Society of America, 88,* 2743–2754.

Bilger, R. C., & Hirsh, I. J. (1956). Masking of tones by bands of noise. *Journal of the Acoustical Society of America, 28,* 623–630.

Boettcher, F., Henderson, D., Gratton, M., Danielson, R., & Byrne, C. (1987). Synergistic interactions of noise and other ototraumatic agents. *Ear and Hearing, 8,* 192–212.

Bohne, B. A. (1976). Safe level for noise exposure? *Annals of Otology, Rhinology, and Laryngology, 85,* 711–724.

Borg, E., Canlon, B., & Engström, B. (1995). Noise-induced hearing loss: Literature review and experiments in rabbits. *Scandinavian Audiology, Suppl. 40.*

Borg, E., & Counter, S. A. (1989). The middle-ear muscles. *Scientific American, 260*(8), 74–80.

Borg, E., Counter, S. A., & Rosler, G. (1984). Theories of the middle-ear muscle function. In S. Silman (Ed.), *The acoustic reflex: Basic principles and clinical applications.* New York: Academic Press.

Borg, E., Nilsson, R., & Engström, B. (1983). Effect of the acoustic reflex on inner ear damage induced by industrial noise. *Acta Otolaryngologica (Stockh.), 96,* 361–369.

Botsford, J. H. (1973). How to estimate dBA reduction of ear protectors. *Journal of Sound and Vibration, 6,* 32–33.

Bronzaft, A. L. (1991). The effects of noise on learning, cognitive development, and social behavior. In T. H. Fay (Ed.), *Noise and Health* (pp. 87–92). New York: The New York Academy of Medicine.

Bronzaft, , A.L., & McCarthy, D.P. (1975). The effect of elevated train noise on reading ability. *Environment and Behavior, 7,* 517–528.

Burns, W., & Robinson, , D. W. (1970). *Hearing and noise in industry.* London: Her Majesty's Stationary Office.

Caiazzo, A., & Tonndorf, J. (1977). Ear canal resonance and temporary threshold shift. *Journal of the Acoustical Society of America, 61,* 578.

Carlin, M. F., & McCrosky, R. L. (1980). Is the eye color a predictor of noise induced hearing loss? *Ear and Hearing, 1,* 191–196.

Carter, N. L. (1980). Eye color and susceptibility to noise induced permanent threshold shift. *Audiology, 19,* 86–93.

CCH Canadian Limited. (1999). *Canadian employment safety and health guide.* Don Mills, ON: CCH Canadian.

Chasin, M. (1989). *The use of the Valsalva maneuver in some musicians to protect hearing.* Technical paper presented at the Ontario Association for Speech-Language Pathologists and Audiologists (OSLA), Toronto, Canada.

Chasin, M. (1994). The acoustic advantages of CIC hearing aids. *Hearing Journal, 47*(11), 13–17.

Chasin, M. (1996). *Musicians and the prevention of hearing loss.* San Diego: Singular Publishing Group.

Chasin, M., & Chong, J. (1992). A clinically efficient hearing protection program for musicians. *Medical Problems of Performing Artists, 7,* 40–43.

Chung, D. Y., Wilson, G. N., Gannon, P., & Mason, K. (1982). Individual susceptibility to noise. In R. P. Hamernik, D. Henderson, & R. Salvi (Eds.), *New perspectives in noise-induced hearing loss* (pp. 511–519). New York: Raven Press.

Clark, W. (1991a). Recent studies of temporary threshold shift (TTS) and permanent threshold shift (PTS) in animals. *Journal of the Acoustical Society of America, 90,* 155–163.

Clark, W. (1991b). Noise exposure from leisure activities: A review. *Journal of the Acoustical Society of America, 90,* 175–181.

Cohen, S., Glass, D., & Singer, J. (1973). Apartment noise, auditory discrimination and reading ability in children. *Journal of Experimental Social Psychology, 9,* 422–437.

Cohen, S., & Weinstein, N. (1981). Non-auditory effects of noise on behavior and health. *The Journal of Social Issues, 37,* 36–70.

Coles, R. R. A. (1987). Tinnitus and its management. In S. D. G. Stephens & A. G. Kerr (Eds.), *Scott Brown's otolaryngology: Audiology* (Vol. 2, 5th ed., pp. 368–414). London: Butterworth.

Cooper, J. C. (1994). Health and nutrition examination survey of 1971–75: Part I. Ear and race effects in hearing. *Journal of the American Academy of Audiology, 5,* 30–36.

Crow, S., Guild, S., & Polvogot, L. (1934). Observation on pathology of high-tone deafness. *Johns Hopkins Medical Journal, 54,* 315–318.

Cudworth, A. L. (1986). Worker's compensation. In E. H. Berger, W. D. Ward, J. C. Morrill, & L. H. Royster, (Eds.), *Noise and hearing conservation manual.* Fairfax, VA: American Industrial Hygiene Association.

Davis, H., Morgan, C. T., Hawkins, J. T., Galambos, R., & Smith, F. W. (1950). Temporary deafness following exposure to loud tones and noise. *Acta Otolaryngologica, 88*(Suppl. 195), 1–57.

Davis, J. (1985). [Hard of hearing children in the schools]. Seminar presentation in St. Cloud, MN.

Dear, T. A. (1998). 5 dB(A): The appropriate exchange rate for workplace noise regulations. *Journal of Occupational Hearing Loss, 1,* 25–37.

DeJoy, D. M. (1984). The nonauditory effects of noise: Review and perspectives for research. *Journal of Auditory Research, 24,* 123–150.

Dengerink, H. A., Lindgren, F., Axelsson, A., & Dengerink, J. E. (1987). The effects of smoking and physical exercise on temporary threshold shifts. *Scandinavian Audiology, 16,* 131–136.

Dengerink, H. A., Trueblood, G. W., & Dengerink, J. E. (1984). The effects of smoking and environmental temperature on temporary threshold shifts. *Audiology, 23,* 401–410.

Edmonds, L. D., Layde, P. M., & Erikson, J. D. (1979). Airport noise and teratogenesis. *Archives of Environmental Health, 34,* 243–247.

Embleton, T. (1995). Upper limits on noise in the workplace. Report by the International Institute of Noise Control Engineering Working Party. *Canadian Acoustics, 23*(2), 11–20.

Environmental Protection Agency. (1973). *Public health and welfare criteria for noise* (EPA Rep. No. 550/9-73-002). Washington, DC: Author.

Fletcher, H., & Munson, W. A. (1933). Loudness, its definition, measurement and calculation. *Journal of the Acoustical Society of America, 5*, 82–108.

Frese, M., & Harwich, C. (1984). Shiftwork and the length and quality of sleep. *Journal of Occupational Medicine, 26*, 561–566.

Gauthier, E., & Burak, M. (1983). Towards a high fidelity hearing aid: The folded horn. *Hearing Aid Journal, 36*(10), 37–39.

Glorig, A., & Linthicum, F. E. (1998). The relations of noise-induced hearing loss and presbycusis. *Journal of Occupational Hearing Loss, 1*, 51–60.

Goldwyn, B., Khan, M. J., Shivapuja, B. G., Seidman, M. D., & Quirk, W. S. (1998). Sarathan preserves cochlear microcirculation and reduces temporary threshold shifts after noise exposure. *Otolaryngology—Head and Neck Surgery, 118*, 576–583.

Green, K. B., Paternak, B. S., & Shore, R. E. (1982). Effects of aircraft noise on reading ability of school-age children. *Archives of Environmental Health, 37*, 24–31.

Guinan, J. J. (1986). Effect of efferent neural activity on cochlear mechanics. In G. Cianfrone & F. Grandori (Eds.), *Cochlear mechanics and otoacoustic emissions* (pp. 53–62). *Scandinavian Audiology*, Suppl. 25.

Hamernik, R. P., & Ahroon, W. A. (1998). Interrupted noise exposures: Threshold shift dynamics and permanent effects. *Journal of the Acoustical Society of America, 103*(6), 3478–3488.

Hawkins, J. E. (1971). The role of vasoconstriction in noise-induced hearing loss. *Annals of Otology, Rhinology, and Laryngology, 80*, 903–913.

Hazell, J., Jastreboff, P. J., Meerton, L. E., & Conway, M. J. (1993). Electrical tinnitus suppression: Frequency dependence of effects. *Audiology, 32*, 68–77.

Health and Welfare Canada. (1987). *Guideline for regulatory control of occupational noise exposure and hearing conservation:* Part I—Model regulation.

Henderson, D., Hamernik, R. P., & Sitler, R. W. (1974). Audiometric and histological correlates of exposure to 1-ms noise impulses in the chinchilla. *Journal of the Acoustical Society of America, 56*, 1210–1221.

Henderson, D., & Saunders, S. S. (1998). Acquisition of noise-induced hearing loss by railway workers. *Ear and Hearing, 19*, 120–130.

Henderson, D., Subramaniam, M., & Boettcher, F. A. (1993). Individual susceptibility to noise-induced hearing loss: An old topic revisited. *Ear and Hearing, 14*, 152–168.

Henselman, L. W., Henderson, D., Shadoan, J., Subramaniam, M., Saunders, S., & Ohlin, D. (1995). Effects of noise exposure, race, and years of service on hearing in U.S. Army soldiers. *Ear and Hearing, 16*, 382–391.

Hétu, R., Phaneuf, R., & Marien, C. (1987). Non-acoustic environmental factor influences on occupational hearing impairment: A preliminary discussion paper. *Canadian Acoustics, 15*(1), 17–31.

Hilding, A. C. (1953). Studies on otic labyrinth: Anatomic explanation for hearing dip at 4096 Hz characteristic of acoustic trauma and presbycusis. *Annals of Otology, Rhinology, and Laryngology, 62*, 950.

Hirsh, I. J., & Bowman, W. D. (1953). Masking of speech by bands of noise. *Journal of the Acoustical Society of America, 25*, 1175–1180.

International Organization for Standardization. (1990). *Acoustics—determination of occupational noise exposure and estimation of noise-induced hearing impairment* (2nd ed). International Standard ISO 1999. Geneva, Switzerland: Author.

Ismail, A. H., Corrigan, D. L., MacLeod, D. F., Anderson, V. L., Kasten, R. N., & Elliot, P. W. (1973). Biophysiological and audiological variables in adults. *Archives of Otolaryngology, 97*, 447–451.

Jastreboff, P. J., & Hazell, J. (1993). A neurophysiological approach to tinnitus: Clinical implications. *British Journal of Audiology, 27*, 7–17.

Jerger, J. F., Tillman, T. W., & Peterson, J. L. (1960). Masking by octave bands of noise in normal and impaired ears. *Journal of the Acoustical Society of America, 32*, 385–390.

Johnson, D. L. (1973). *Prediction of NIPTS due to continuous noise exposure* (Aerospace Medical Research Laboratory Report Number AMRL-TR-73-91), Dayton, OH: Wright-Patterson Air Force Base.

Johnson, D. L. (1991). Field studies: Industrial exposures. *Journal of the Acoustical Society of America, 90*, 170–174.

Johnson, D. L., & Nixon, C. W. (1974). Simplified methods for estimating hearing protector performance. *Journal of Sound and Vibration, 7*, 20–27.

Johnson, R. M., Brummet, R., & Schleuning, A. (1993). Use of Aprazolam for relief of tinnitus. *Archives of Otolaryngology—Head and Neck Surgery, 119*, 842–845.

Killion, M. C. (1993). The parvum bonum, plus melius fallacy in earplug selection. In L. Beilin & G. R. Jensen (Eds.), *Recent developments in hearing instrument technology* (15th Danavox Symposium) (pp. 415–433). Kolding, Denmark: Scanticon. [The Danavox Jubilee Foundation.]

Killion, M. C., DeVilbiss, E., & Stewart, J. (1988). An earplug with uniform 15-dB attenuation. *Hearing Journal, 41*(5), 14–16.

Killion, M. C., Stewart, J. K., Falco, R., & Berger, E. H. (1992). *Improved audibility earplug*. U.S. Patent 5,113,967.

Knox, A. W. (1993). Tinnitus: A review of the literature. *Spectrum* (The National Hearing Conservation Association Newsletter), *10*(1), 1–9.

Kryter, K. D., Ward, W. D., Miller, J. D., & Eldredge, D. H. (1966). Hazardous exposures to intermittent and steady-state noise. *Journal of the Acoustical Society of America, 39*, 451–464.

Langendorf, F. G. (1992). Absolute pitch: Review and speculations. *Medical Problems of Performing Artists, 7*(1), 6–13.

Lawrence, M., Gonzales, G., & Hawkins, J. E. (1967). Some physiological factors in noise induced hearing loss. *American Industrial Hygiene Journal, 28*, 425–428.

Lempert, B. L., & Henderson, T. L. (1973). NIOSH survey of occupational noise and hearing: 1968 to 1972. Washington, DC: U.S. Department of Health, Education and Welfare, National Institute for Occupational Safety and Health, TR 86.

Levine, R. A. (1994). Tinnitus. *Current Opinion in Otolaryngology and Head and Neck Surgery, 2*, 171–176.

Lim, D. J. (1986). Cochlear micromechanics in understanding otoacoustic emission. In G. Cianfrone & F. Grandori (Eds.), *Cochlear mechanics and otoacoustic emissions* (pp. 17–26). *Scandinavian Audiology*, (Suppl. 25).

Lonsbury-Martin, B. L., Harris, F. P., Hawkins, M. D., Stagner, B. B., & Martin, G. K. (1990). Distortion product emissions in humans II: Relations to acoustic immittance and stimulus frequency and spontaneous otoacoustic emissions in normally hearing subjects. *Annals of Otology, Rhinology, and Laryngology, 147*(Suppl. 99), 15–28.

Macrae, J. H. (1991). Presbycusis and noise-induced permanent threshold shift. *Journal of the Acoustical Society of America, 90*, 2513–2516.

Mahoney, C. F. O., & Kemp, D. (1995). Distortion product otoacoustic emission delay measurements in human ears. *Journal of the Acoustical Society of America, 97*, 3721–3735.

Martin, A. (1976). The equal energy concept applied to impulse noise. In D. Henderson, R. P. Hamernik, D. S. Dosanjh, & J. H. Mills (Eds.), *Effects of noise on hearing* (pp. 421–453). New York: Raven Press.

Martin, F. N., Champlin, C. A., & Chambers, J. A. (1998). Seventh survey of audiometric practices in the United States. *Journal of the American Academy of Audiology, 9*, 95–104.

Matkin, N. (1988). [Changing characteristics and the implications to clinical and educational services in the hearing impaired child]. Seminar presentation in Minneapolis, MN.

Melnick, W. (1991). Human temporary threshold shift (TTS) and damage risk. *Journal of the Acoustical Society of America, 90*, 147–154.

Miller, J. D., Watson, C. S., & Covell, W. P. (1963). Deafening effects of noise on the cat. *Acta Otolaryngologica*(Supp. 176), 1–91.

Mills, J. H., Boettcher, F. A., & Dubno, J. R. (1997). Interaction of noise-induced permanent threshold shift and age-related threshold shift. *Journal of the Acoustical Society of America, 101*, 1681–1686.

Mills, J. H., Gilbert, R. M., & Adkins, W. Y. (1979). Temporary threshold shifts in humans exposed to octave bands of noise for 16 to 24 hours. *Journal of the Acoustical Society of America, 65*, 1238–1248.

Mills, J. H., Osguthorpe, J. D., Burdick, C. K., Patterson, J. H., & Mozo, B. (1983). Temporary threshold shifts produced by exposure to low-frequency noises. *Journal of the Acoustical Society of America, 73*, 918–923.

Miyakita, T., Hellstrom, P. A., Frimansson, E., & Axelsson, A. (1992). Effect of low level acoustic stimulation on temporary threshold shift in young humans. *Hearing Research, 60*, 149–155.

Murai, K., Tyler, R. S., Harker, L. A., & Stouffer, J. L. (1992). Review of pharmacologic treatment of tinnitus. *American Journal of Otology, 13*, 454–464.

Nakamura, R. (1977). Gestation and noise [Abstract]. In S. Toongsuwan & T. Suvonnakoto (Eds.), Congress Handbook, Seventh Asian Congress of Obstetrics and Gynecology, Bangkok, Thailand.

National Institute for Occupational Safety and Health (NIOSH), U.S. Department of Health, Education, and Welfare. (1973). Occupational noise and hearing 1968–1972. HSM 73-11001. Washington, DC: NIOSH.

Nixon, C. W., Hille, H. K., & Kettler, L. K. (1967). *Attenuation characteristics of earmuffs at low audio and infrasonic frequencies.* Rep. AMRL-TR-67-27. Dayton, OH. Wright-Patterson Air Force Base.

OSHA. (1983). Occupational noise exposure: Hearing conservation amendment; Final Rule. *Federal Register, 48*, 9738–9785.

Passchier-Vermeer, W. (1968). Hearing loss due to exposure to steady-state broadband noise (Rep. No. 35). The Netherlands: Institute for Public Health Engineering.

Passchier-Vermeer, W. (1971). Steady-state and fluctuating noise: Its effects on the hearing of people. In D. W. Robinson (Ed.), *Occupational hearing loss*. New York: Academic Press.

Patchett, R. (1992). The effects of inhalation of oxygen and carbon dioxide mixtures on noise-induced temporary threshold shift in humans. *Canadian Acoustics, 20*(1), 21–25.

Pickett, J. M. (1959). Low-frequency noise and methods for calculating speech intelligibility. *Journal of the Acoustical Society of America, 31*, 1259–1263.

Pollak, C. (1991). The effects of noise on sleep. In T. H. Fay (Ed.), *Noise & health* (pp. 41–60). New York: The New York Academy of Medicine.

Preves, D. A., & Pehringer, J. L. (1983). Calculating individuals NRRs in situ using subminiature probe microphones. *Hearing Instruments, 33*(3), 10–14.

Price, G. R. (1994). *Occasional exposure to impulsive sounds: Significant noise exposure?* Forum presented at the 19th annual National Hearing Conservation Association (NHCA) Conference, Atlanta, GA.

Price, G. R., & Kalb, J. T. (1991). Insights into hazard from intense impulses from a mathematical model of the ear. *Journal of the Acoustical Society of America, 90*, 219–227.

Prince, M. M., & Matonoski, G. M. (1991). Problems on ascertaining the combined effects of exposure: Results of an occupational cohort study of the joint effects of noise and smoking on hearing acuity. In L. Fechter (Ed.), *Proceedings of the IVth international conference on the combined effects of environmental factors* (pp. 87–91). Baltimore: Johns Hopkins University Press.

Raymond, L. W. (1991). Neuroendocrine, immunologic, and gastointestinal effects of noise. In T. H. Fay (Ed.), *Noise & Health* (pp. 27–40). New York: The New York Academy of Medicine.

Robinson, D. W. (1968). *The relationship between hearing loss and noise exposure*. National Physical Laboratory Aero Rep. Ae32. London: England: National Physical Laboratory.

Robinson, D. W. (1971). Estimating the risk of hearing loss due to continuous noise. In D. W. Robinson (Ed.) *Occupational hearing loss*. New York: Academic Press.

Robinson, D. W. (1976). Characteristics of occupational noise-induced hearing loss. In D. Henderson, R. P. Hamernik, D. S. Dosanjh, & J. H. Mills (Eds.), *Effects of noise on hearing*. New York: Raven Press.

Robinson, D. W. (1988). Threshold of hearing as a function of age and sex for the typical unscreened population. *British Journal of Audiology, 22*(1), 5–20.

Rosenhall, U., Pedersen, K., & Svanborg, A. (1990). Presbycusis and noise-induced hearing loss. *Ear and Hearing, 11*, 257–263.

Rosowski, J. (1991). The effects of external- and middle-ear filtering on auditory threshold and noise-induced hearing loss. *Journal of the Acoustical Society of America, 90*, 124–135.

Royster, J. D., and Royster, L. H. (1994). Practical tips for fitting hearing protection. *Hearing Instruments, 45*, 17–18.

Ryals, B. M. (1990). Critical periods and acoustic trauma. In *National Institutes of Health (NIH) Consensus Development Conference on Noise and Hearing Loss. Program and Abstracts.* Washington, DC.

Sanden, A., & Axelsson, A. (1981). Comparison of cardiovascular responses in noise-resistant and noise-sensitive workers. *Acta Otolaryngologica (Stockh.), 76*(Suppl. 377), 75–100.

Sataloff, R. T., & Sataloff, J. (1993). *Occupational hearing loss.* New York: Marcel Dekker.

Schell, L. M. (1981). Environmental noise and human prenatal growth. *American Journal of Physical Anthropology, 56,* 156–163.

Schroeter, J. (1986). The use of acoustical test fixtures for the measurement of hearing protector attenuation. Part I: Review of previous work and the design of an improved test fixture. *Journal of the Acoustical Society of America, 79,* 1065–1081.

Schuknecht, H., & Tonndorf, J. (1960). Acoustic trauma of the cochlea from ear surgery. *Laryngoscope, 70,* 479.

Selters, W., & Ward, W. D. (1962). Temporary threshold shift with changing duty cycles. *Journal of the Acoustical Society of America, 34,* 122–123.

Shaw, E. A .G., & Theissen, G. J. (1958). Improved cushion for ear defenders. *Journal of the Acoustical Society of America, 30,* 24–36.

Shaw, E. A. G., & Theissen, G. J. (1962). Acoustics of circumaural earphones. *Journal of the Acoustical Society of America, 34,* 1233–1243.

Sivan, L. J., & White, S. D. (1933). On minimum audible fields. *Journal of the Acoustical Society of America, 4,* 288–321.

Sloan, R. P. (1991). Cardiovascular effects of noise. In T. H. Fay (Ed.), *Noise & health* (pp. 15–26). New York: The New York Academy of Medicine.

Smith, E. L., & Laird, D. A. (1930). The loudness of auditory stimuli which affect stomach contractions in healthy human beings. *Journal of the Acoustical Society of America, 15,* 94–98.

Spoendlin, H. (1986). Receptoneural and innervation aspects of the inner ear anatomy with respect to cochlear mechanics. In G. Cianfrone & F. Grandori (Eds.), *Cochlear mechanics and otoacoustic emissions* (pp. 27–34). *Scandinavian Audiology,* (Suppl. 25).

Stevens, S. S. (1961). Procedure for calculating loudness. *Journal of the Acoustical Society of America, 33,* 1577–1585.

Subramaniam, M., Henderson, D., & Spongr, V. (1991). Frequency differences in the development of protection against NIHL by low level "toughening" exposures. *Journal of the Acoustical Society of America, 89*(4, Part 2), 1865–1874.

Swanson, S. J., Dengerink, H. A., Kondrick, P., & Miller, C. L. (1987). The influence of subjective factors on temporary threshold shifts after exposure to music and noise of equal energy. *Ear and Hearing, 8,* 288–291.

Taylor, W., Pearson, J., Mair, W., & Burns, W. (1965). Study of noise and hearing in jute weaving. *Journal of the Acoustical Society of America, 38,* 113–120.

Thiessen, G. J. (1978). Disturbance of sleep by noise. *Journal of the Acoustical Society of America, 64,* 216–222.

Thiessen, G. J. (1983). Effect of intermittent and continuous traffic noise on various sleep characteristics and their adaptation. In G. Rossi (Ed.), *Proceedings of the Fourth International Congress on Noise as a Public Health Problem (Turin)* (Vol. 2). Milan, Italy: Edizioni Techn021iche a cura del Centro Ricerche e Studi Amplifon.

Thompson, S. J. (1981). Epidemiology feasibility study: Effects of noise on the cardiovascular system. Washington, DC: United States Environmental Protection Agency.

Tonndorf, J. (1976). Relationship between the transmission characteristics of conductive system and noise-induced hearing loss. In D. Henderson, R. P. Hamernik, D. S. Dosanjh, & J. H. Mills (Eds.) *Effects of noise on hearing* (pp. 159–178). New York: Raven Press.

Tyler, R. S., Aran, J-M., & Dauman, R. (1992, November). Recent advances in tinnitus. *American Journal of Audiology*, pp. 36–43.

United States Department of Labor, Occupational Safety and Health Administration. (1981). Occupational noise exposure: hearing conservation amendment, Part III. *Federal Register, 46*, 4078–4179.

Vittitow, M., Windmill, I. M., Yates, J. W., & Cunningham, D. R. (1994). Effect of simultaneous exercise and noise exposure (music) on hearing. *Journal of the American Academy of Audiology, 5*, 343–348.

Wachs, T. D. (1982). *Relation of home noise-confusion to infant cognitive development.* Paper presented at the Annual Meeting of the American Psychological Association, Washington, DC.

Ward, W. D. (1970). Temporary threshold shift and damage risk criteria for intermittent noise exposures. *Journal of the Acoustical Society of America, 48*, 561–574.

Ward, W. D. (1974). Noise levels are not noise exposures! *Proceedings of NOIS-EXPO Conference*, 170–175.

Ward, W. D. (1976). A comparison of the effects of continuous, intermittent and impulse noise. In D. Henderson, R. P. Hamernik, D. S. Dosanjh, & J. H. Mills (Eds.), *Effects of noise on hearing* (pp. 407–420). New York: Raven Press.

Ward, W. D. (1982). Summation of international symposium on hearing protection in industry. In P. A. Alberti (Ed.), *Personal hearing protection in industry* (pp. 577–592). New York: Raven Press.

Ward, W. D. (1991). The role of intermittence in PTS. *Journal of the Acoustical Society of America, 90*, 164–169.

Ward, W. D., Cushing, E. M., & Burns, E. M. (1976). Effective quiet and moderate TTS: Implications for noise exposure standards. *Journal of the Acoustical Society of America, 59*, 160–165.

Ward, W. D. (1998). Presbycusis and NIHL: Current DRC and the validity of EEH noise susceptibility and new psychoacoustic methods. *Journal of Occupational Hearing Loss, 1*, 17–24.

Zakrisson, J-E, Borg, E., Liden, G., & Nilsson, R. (1980). Stapedius reflex in industrial impact noise: Fatigability and role for temporary threshold shift (TTS). *Scandinavian Audiology*, (Suppl. 12), 326–334.

Zheng, X. Y., Henderson, D., McFadden, S. L., & Hu, B. H. (1997). The role of the cochlear efferent system in acquired resistance to noise-induced hearing loss. *Hearing Research, 104*, 191–203.

Zwislocki, J. (1953). Acoustic attenuation between the ears. *Journal of the Acoustical Society of America, 25,* 752–759.

Zwislocki, J. (1957). In search of the bone-conduction threshold in a free sound field. *Journal of the Acoustical Society of America, 29,* 795–804.

Index